MW01181145

Provider
Report
Cards

A Guide for Promoting Health Care
Quality to the Public

Patrice L. Spath, Editor

Health Forum, Inc.
An American Hospital Association Company
CHICAGO

AHA
press

Printed in the United States of America—3/99

Cover design by Dan Stein

ISBN: 1-55648-250-7

Item number: 136112

*This book is dedicated to Donald M. Berwick, MD,
a man who is genuinely committed to improving
the quality of health care services for all patients.*

Contents

CHAPTER FIVE

Developing and Disseminating the Michigan
Hospital Report   *75*

Mark Sonneborn, MS, CHE

PART TWO
Measuring Provider Performance

CHAPTER SIX

Gathering Satisfaction Data to Share with the Public   *97*

J. Mac Crawford, RN, MS, PhD, and John F. Sena, PhD

CHAPTER SEVEN

*Assessing How Provider Health Care Programs Enhance
Community Quality of Life*   *119*

Don R. Rahtz, PhD, and M. Joseph Sirgy, PhD

About the Authors

EDITOR

Patrice L. Spath, BA, ART, a health care quality specialist based in Forest Grove, Oregon, has extensive experience in quality and resource management initiatives. She was previously a regional councilor for the Health Care Division of the American Society for Quality and chair of the Quality Management Section of the American Health Information Management Association (AHIMA). A much sought–after speaker, she has presented more than 350 educational programs on performance improvement, case management, utilization review, clinical paths, and outcomes management. She is the author of several books, video programs, and journal articles on these subjects. For AHA Press she was the editor of *Clinical Paths: Tools for Outcomes Management,* published in 1994; *Medical Effectiveness and Outcomes Management: Issues, Methods, and Case Studies,* published in 1996; and *Beyond Clinical Paths: Advanced Tools for Outcomes Management,* published in 1997. Information about her other publications can be found at her Web site at www.brownspath.com.

Ms. Spath is a regular columnist for *Hospital Peer Review* and *Hospital Case Management* and is editor for *The Quality Resource,* the newsletter of the Quality Management Section of the AHIMA. She served on a work group of the Agency for Health Care Policy and Research to assist in the development of a model for translating its clinical practice guidelines to medical review criteria, performance measures, and standards of quality. She was a member of the Clinical Guidelines Panel of the Veterans Health Administration and a member of the Clinical Path Work Group of the Association of Operating Room Nurses, Inc. Recently, she served as an on-line expert on outcomes management topics for the "Ask the Expert" feature of the *Modern Healthcare* Web site.

AUTHORS

J. Mac Crawford, RN, MS, PhD, is currently in the School of Public Health at The Ohio State University. Formerly, he was director of research at National Research Corporation (NRC). He has been in the health care field for over 20 years, working as an emergency medical technician, nursing assistant, registered nurse, and epidemiologist. His work with NRC included questionnaire design and proofing, data analysis, consulting, teaching within the company, and writing for publication.

Alice G. Gosfield, Esq., practices law in Philadelphia through Alice G. Gosfield and Associates, PC (www.gosfield.com). She has specialized in health law and health care regulation since 1973. She also serves as the board chair of the National Committee for Quality Assurance. She publishes and lectures frequently on health law issues for such groups as the Medical Group Management Association, American Health Lawyers Association, and the American Association of Health Plans. She serves on the editorial boards of several periodicals. She was president of the National Health Lawyers Association from 1992 to 1993. Her second book, *Guide to Key Legal Issues in Managed Care Quality,* was published in 1996 by Faulkner & Gray.

Mary M. Krieg, RN,C, MS, is president and CEO of Quality Management Consultants, Inc. She has more than 20 years of experience in clinical nursing and health care quality improvement and is a nationally recognized expert in the design and implementation of quality improvement projects. She directed implementation of the Health Care Financing Administration's national pilot project, the Cooperative Cardiovascular Project, in Iowa. She has lectured throughout the country on the subject of provider report cards and has written a number of articles. Her "Top Ten List of Quality Indicators" may be found at her Web site: www.iowahealth.net/qmc.

Michelle H. Pelling, MBA, RN, is president of The Propell Group, an Oregon-based consulting firm providing health care management consulting in the areas of service quality/patient satisfaction, consumer-oriented report cards, performance measurement, quality improvement, and team effectiveness. She lectures around the country and has had extensive experience assisting organizations throughout the United States and Canada. She is the author of two books and several journal articles.

Don R. Rahtz, PhD, is associate professor of marketing at The College of William and Mary in Williamsburg, Virginia. He is vice-president for external affairs of the International Society of Quality of Life Studies and was instrumental in its development. He has done substantial research and consulting in the quality of life and health care areas. He holds a PhD in marketing from Virginia Tech and an MBA from Northern Illinois University.

John F. Sena, PhD, was a professor at The Ohio State University for 29 years. He has coauthored, with Stephen Strasser, PhD, three books on career development and is currently writing a book on recent developments in patient-perceived outcome measurements. He is an active lecturer and speaker and has extensive experience conducting focus groups. He has given seminars for the American College of Healthcare Executives for the past eight years.

M. Joseph Sirgy, PhD, is professor of marketing at Virginia Polytechnic Institute and State University and executive director and founder of the International Society of Quality of Life Studies. He is director of the office of Quality-of-Life Measurement (http://www.cob.st.edu/market/center1.htm). He has done extensive research, writing, and consulting in the health care field in relation to community quality of life.

Mark Sonneborn, MS, CHE, is senior director, data and quality initiatives, for the Michigan Health & Hospital Association. He is responsible for coordinating the production of the *Michigan Hospital Report,* an annual publication with hospital-specific performance information (www.mha.org). He is also a project manager for other MHA public reporting initiatives.

Charles E. Swain is a principal with the Internet development and consulting company CSEnterprises and actively supports the Internet operations of several health care consulting firms. He is affiliated with Swain & Associates, a St. Petersburg health care consulting firm, as an educator and project manager (www.snaconsulting.com). Mr. Swain has been responsible for designing and implementing voice and data telecommunications networks for a large transportation company, developed methods to assist organizations in their improvement efforts, and trained health care providers in how to develop skills in Internet searching, benchmarking, and quality management. He is active in the Florida Association of Healthcare Quality, Area II, and contributes Internet expertise to other professional health care organizations.

Foreword

As president of the Society for Healthcare Consumer Advocacy (SHCA), a personal membership group of the American Hospital Association, I represent the ideals and goals of an organization of over 1,050 health care consumer advocates. These dedicated professionals work diligently to assist health care consumers in making informed decisions with regard to their health care regimen. SHCA members can be found throughout the industry. In Canada and the United States, from hospitals to nursing homes, from HMOs to other forms of managed care, we subscribe to a basic vision: *Empower the health care consumer with knowledge to make informed decisions and restore consumer trust in the health care system and the delivery of the service.*

Seemingly simplistic goals. Are they reachable? Are they realistic? It is every health care organization's responsibility to make those answers affirmative. I would also support these as the goals of all health care professionals.

The consumer must be empowered! Knowledge is an influential tool. An uneducated consumer runs the risk of accepting decisions that may be ill advised. How could it be otherwise?

Without the informed consumer, the system cannot function smoothly. Without a smoothly functioning system, public cynicism about the health care system will flourish and the very delivery of health care suffers.

The key to reaching the lofty perch of consumer empowerment is information. This information must be accurate and timely. Most important, the information must be understandable to the consumer, and it must be reliable. Has it been researched? If so, does it have application to consumers? We are in the information age, we are getting more information all the time, and it is coming more quickly, creating, many times, *system overload!*

Those of us involved in the delivery of the health care experience have an obligation. We must assimilate a mountain of knowledge, find the very best information we can that is applicable, and put it into terms consumers can understand. Again, this sounds simple, but it doesn't happen as often or as well as it should. Health care consumers are beginning to demand the empowerment of knowledge. They may not know exactly what it is they *need* to know, but they *demand* to know. Educate them and make them active participants in their own treatment, not merely recipients of assigned procedures.

What do providers know that is important for patients to know? If you ask consumers what they want to know, they'll tell you. But you've got to ask. Patients are dealing with enough—illness, anxiety, and even fear. They need confidence in providers and the system. Acknowledging their concerns and fears and addressing questions with accuracy will promote trust and confidence among your consumers. Ultimately, confidence that the provider is really concerned will become confidence in the system. By listening, you know what they want to know. You must fill in the blanks at times, tell them *what* they need to know and *why* they need to know it.

Moreover, consumers are becoming aware that benchmarks exist. Many are making health care provider decisions based on a certain institution's track record. The benchmarks offer a "compare and contrast study" of sorts. Indeed, some consumers choose their providers because of convenience or familiarity. But more and more, they are basing their "provider of choice" decisions on patient outcomes, duration of stay, and quality of treatment. In other words, they have been empowered by knowledge to choose, and they are exercising that right.

This book is a piece of the puzzle in reaching our goal for educating consumers. It will provide the tools to develop and implement a plan to provide health care consumers with the information they need to make truly informed and participatory decisions concerning their health care, which in turn affects their health. It is not much of a reach to say that an informed consumer has the opportunity to make better health choices. It would stand to reason, then, that the result is an opportunity for better health. Isn't that what we're all here for? Isn't that the ultimate goal?

Diana P. Tuell
Director of Patient Relations
Central Baptist Hospital, Lexington, KY

1998 President of the Society for Healthcare Consumer Advocacy of the American Hospital Association

Preface

Activities designed to evaluate the quality of health care services have been in existence for several decades. However, the specific results of these activities have been kept confidential. Other than through personal attestations or knowing that an organization was accredited or licensed, until recently purchasers and the public had no way of knowing which organization provided the best health care.

Health plans were the first to publish information about performance. These publications were originally referred to in the news media as "report cards," and that title has persisted. Performance measures in these report cards included items such as mammography rates, immunization rates, lung cancer survival rates, results of patient satisfaction surveys, and claims turnaround time. Health plan performance measurement data were intended to be used by employers to select health plans offering the greatest value and by providers to determine which health plans they wanted to associate with. Presumably, the public would use health plan report cards in making choices among health plan offerings.

More recently, health care providers have begun to create their own quality report cards to publicize superior performance to purchasers, health plans, and consumers themselves. Provider performance report cards can include both clinical and administrative performance measures, such as mortality rates for patients who had surgery, cancer survival rates, patient satisfaction data, number of board-certified physicians, lengths of hospital stay, and charges for certain conditions.

There remain many obstacles to creating the ideal health care report card, whether it be a health plan report or one created by a provider. These difficulties include the following:

- Inaccurate, misleading, or incomplete information sources
- Indicators that may not measure quality as defined by the various users of the report
- Little agreement on formulas for calculating performance results
- Little or no verification mechanisms in place to ensure the accuracy of reported results
- Lack of standardized patient satisfaction survey instruments
- Less than adequate understanding of what information is most useful to the public
- Conflicting opinions on how best to design consumer-oriented report cards and how the reports should be made available

The public, however, has little understanding of the report card issues that payers and providers continue to grapple with. Most consumers are not concerned about the complexities of developing valid and reliable health care measures. Recent studies indicate that consumers are primarily troubled about rising out-of-pocket expenses, freedom of provider choice, and the impact of managed care on quality. Nonetheless, regulators, payers, and providers themselves are seeking better ways to educate consumers on how to measure health care quality and judge the value of services they are receiving.

"People spend much more time using their *Consumer Reports, Motor Trend,* or *Auto Week* when they buy a new car than they ever spend thinking about whether they have the right doctor. Or when they're at that doctor's office, are they having the right decisions made," said Peter Lee of the Center for Health Care Rights in Los Angeles. Is the reason for consumers' seeming lack of interest in health care performance data due to the unavailability of objective and consumer-friendly comparative information? If such information is made available, will it be read? Are the health care industry and its external regulators championing report card initiatives that will end up disregarded by the vast majority of health care consumers? Only the passage of time will reveal the answers to these questions.

Health care performance data are of interest to a variety of audiences, including purchasers (private and governmental) who want to ensure accountability for quality and the data needed to guide purchasing decisions and providers themselves who want information for internal quality improvement and to use in marketing quality to purchasers and consumers. As consumers shoulder more personal responsibility for health care expenses, they want information to guide their purchasing decisions (when choosing a health plan and/or personal caregivers).

This book is intended to clarify what consumers need to know in order to choose a provider. Within the context of this book, *consumer* refers to all potential individual end users of health care (i.e., men, women, and children who receive the health services delivered by physicians, nurses, dentists, and other licensed and unlicensed health care providers). A *provider* is considered to be any organization or individual involved in the provision of direct patient care. A *report card* is a description of performance that includes one or more measures that are intended to communicate to consumers the quality characteristics of a provider. The definition of quality from a consumer standpoint continues to be debated.

This book is divided into two parts. The first part, "Designing and Disseminating Provider Report Cards," consists of five chapters. Chapter 1 addresses the concept of "quality" as defined by the public. For consumer-oriented provider report cards to be useful, they must contain information that answers questions of interest to the public. The authors of this chapter explore this issue by presenting results from recent studies that asked people what is important to them when choosing a provider. Chapter 2 describes what providers must do to develop and distribute a report card to the public. The authors outline a framework for discussing the important elements of measurement selection, data presentation, and dissemination. Also included in this chapter is a checklist of design and dissemination considerations.

The Internet has become an important provider communication link with consumers. Today, more than 25,000 health care-related Web sites can be accessed by anyone with a telephone line and a personal computer. An Internet-based dissemination strategy is fast becoming a critical element in providers' efforts to share performance data with consumers. Chapter 3 provides an overview of the issues related to Web site design and tips on how to create a consumer-friendly Internet-based report card.

With performance data now being shared with the public, concerns about the legal perils are surfacing. Chapter 4 addresses these worries by outlining the legal issues most likely to arise and some commonsense tips for avoiding trouble when creating provider report cards. Chapter 5 describes the steps taken by the Michigan Health & Hospital Association in creating the *Michigan Hospital Report*. This chapter provides important insights into the process of report card development and the decisions that must be made during the design and distribution stages.

The second part of this book, "Measuring Provider Performance," deals with two important measures of provider performance: patient satisfaction and community contributions. These quality characteristics are likely to be very high on the list of what consumers want to know about health care organizations. Chapter 6 outlines a framework for collecting patient satisfaction data that can be communicated to the public. This chapter includes practical tips for gathering satisfaction ratings that are useful for both internal performance improvement and external reporting. Health care organizations play an important role in community wellness, and the authors of chapter 7 describe a unique model for measuring the impact of provider services on community quality of life. The measurement activities create a one-of-a-kind opportunity for health care providers to partner with their community in improving the social well-being of consumers.

This book contains up-to-date information about consumer-oriented, provider-generated report cards. Whether these report cards are viewed as valuable educational tools by consumers has yet to be adequately judged. It is unlikely, however, that the health care industry will ever again see the pre-report-card environment. Signs of the growth of health care consumerism are everywhere. Providers cannot sit back and wait until the researchers resolve the complex issues of performance measurement. Although we may not be totally satisfied with today's quality ratings and available distribution methods, it is imperative that providers assume a leadership role in communicating quality to the public.

Acknowledgments

The fine authors represented in this book deserve a hearty thanks for sharing their vast knowledge and experiences. A person who also deserves special thanks is Judy Homa-Lowry of Canton, Michigan. Her constant encouragement and unwavering faith helped to make this book a success.

Patrice L. Spath, BA, ART
Health Care Quality Specialist
Forest Grove, Oregon

PART ONE

Designing and Disseminating Provider Report Cards

CHAPTER ONE

Determining What Consumers Want to Know about Providers

Michelle H. Pelling, MBA, RN
Patrice L. Spath, BA, ART

The content of health care provider-specific report cards must be based on the adage, "The customer is king." However, after more than ten years of experience with performance reports, we are still grappling with the issue of what to include in reports intended for the general public. Providers tell the public: "These are the questions you should be asking about your caregivers." Common recommendations are costs, volume, average length of hospital stay (ALOS), and mortality rates. In turn, consumers tell providers they want basic information about access, satisfaction, follow-up, and other measures more difficult to quantify.[1] Although provider-oriented report cards are considered a way to create better-informed consumers, there are few definitive answers about what consumers actually want to know.

This chapter describes various studies that have attempted to answer the questions of how consumers choose health care providers and what attributes consumers consider important in making their choices. It also discusses information that providers might include in the report cards intended for the public.

Factors That Influence When Consumers Seek Information about Providers

Uwe Reinhardt, a nationally recognized expert on health economics and policy, suggests that consumers do not think much about health care when they are healthy.[2] He draws a significant distinction between information the general public would like to see on provider-specific report cards and what patients might wish to know. He contends that it's only when people become ill and require the services of a physician or hospital that they are able to appreciate the significance of service and clinical outcome measures. His comments are supported by general marketing research suggesting that consumers with a great knowledge of a particular product (experts) process information differently than novices do.[3] Experts (for example, current patients) are likelier to respond to data about intrinsic attributes that pertain to the quality of a product or service, whereas novices (people who sporadically interact with or who have never interacted with the health care delivery system) are likelier to respond to information on the benefits of a particular product or service (for example, availability of after-hours care and lower prices). However, even novices may not be concerned with the cost of health care services if their out-of-pocket expenses are minimal.

Whether consumers will use the information on provider-oriented report cards to select health care providers is uncertain. Consumer decision-making models from the marketing literature suggest that people must first perceive the need for information before they seek out relevant product facts.[4] Likewise, the less financial risk in a purchasing decision, the less effort consumers devote to learning more about the product.

However, recent media coverage of medical errors, adverse drug events, and variations in clinical outcomes is directing consumer attention to the importance of health care quality and creating a perceived need for provider-specific data. As this need becomes ingrained, consumers will demand more facts about the attributes of health care services they consider important when making purchasing decisions. Drawing from the experiences of other industries, health care providers can play an important role in influencing consumer perceptions about what is important. For example, in the 1980s, Burger King persuaded consumers that an important attribute of fast-food hamburgers was the method of cooking—flame broiling.[5] Various organizations have already begun to influence public opinion about what's important in choosing a hospital. For example, the Pacific Business Group on Health recommends that people consider these characteristics when selecting a hospital: accreditation status, types of high-volume procedures, staffing and service capabilities, quality assurance activities, and how patients fared after surgery.[6]

Consumers are important stakeholders in the health care delivery system. Health plans and individual health care organizations are finding that the public can provoke shifts in provider panels and practice patterns when they perceive quality is being compromised.[7,8] For this reason, it is imperative that health care providers understand more about what consumers value.

Factors That Influence Consumer Selection of Providers

Several factors come into play when consumers are in a position to select a provider. These include the following:

- Opinions of friends and family
- Opinions of experts

- Personal attributes of providers
- Provider cost
- Provider demographics

Opinions of Friends and Family

A 1996 national poll sponsored jointly by the Agency for Health Care Policy and Research (AHCPR) and the Kaiser Family Foundation found that when choosing providers, consumers rely primarily on the recommendations of people they know and trust (family, friends, personal physician).[9] A recent project of the SPRY (Setting Priorities for Retirement Years) Foundation investigated how elderly people and their families make decisions about long-term care.[10] Interviews were conducted with 63 elderly individuals and their families who had recently changed their living situations to meet long-term care needs. When asked how they had made their choices, most respondents said they had relied on their physicians for guidance, although many felt their physicians were not as helpful as they would have liked. They also relied heavily on family members or friends for information.

Relying on the opinions of others in the purchasing decision is a common choice when consumer expertise is low. Uninformed consumers tend to replace product evaluation with information source evaluation; that is, they decide whether they trust a given opinion.[11] Until consumers become "experts" in the clinical intricacies of health care, they are likely to continue to rely heavily on the opinions of people they trust. It is important to note that 50 percent of the AHCPR/Kaiser survey respondents indicated that the advice given by friends and family was "very believable," compared with only 7 percent who relied on government-generated information and 5 percent who trusted information obtained from newspapers, television, and other media.

This consumer behavior is common to all industries. In fact, word-of-mouth communication is estimated to account for three times as many purchases as compared to formal advertisements.[12] Consumers are very likely to seek purchasing recommendations from other consumers when they do not believe advertisements, want to decrease their anxiety about making a risky purchase, or when the product is highly complex (for example, health care services). The public appears to want more information about the actual experiences of patients like themselves and how they fared with a particular hospital, physician, or health plan. Levitan and Cleary of the Picker Institute encourage providers to incorporate "word-of-mouth" communications into their report card strategy. They strongly believe that the inclusion of previous patients' experiences with care and their satisfaction levels could increase the usefulness of report card data for consumers.[13] Shoshanna Sofaer, director for the Center of Outcomes Improvement Research, George Washington University, also stresses the importance of providing healthy consumers with information about previous patients' experiences. However, she suggests that in addition to satisfaction data, healthy consumers also want to know how people were treated when they did get sick (for example, was access to care timely? Was specialty care available if needed? Did patients feel they were denied necessary services?).[14]

Opinions of Experts

The opinions of "experts" may also be sought by the uneducated or apprehensive consumer. Generally, these experts fall into the following three categories:

1. People viewed as having firsthand knowledge of the product or service (for example, personal physician, patients, and people employed by the provider)

2. A "surrogate consumer"—one who acts as the consumer's agent to guide, direct, and/or translate complex data (for example, health plan, employer, and federal or state agencies)
3. Impartial consumer advisory groups that offer information about many kinds of products and services (such as *Consumer Reports*)

Personal Attributes of Providers

In the AHCPR/Kaiser survey, consumers were also asked what they thought were the most important attributes influencing their selection of a new doctor. Communication abilities and caring attitude ranked highest in importance; the next highest was evidence of additional training and testing in his or her area of specialty. Habit also appeared to influence consumer decisions. Most survey respondents said they would stick with the provider (surgeon or hospital) they had been satisfied with in the past, even though others may be rated higher in quality by the experts. It appears that if the consumers' decision worked for them in the past, they are less apt to change caregivers based on quality ratings alone.

Provider Cost

Today's health care consumers are cost-sensitive. Findings in the Health Confidence Survey (HCS) conducted in February 1998 by the Employee Benefits Research Institute and Mathew Greenwald & Associates revealed that a large majority of the 1,002 survey participants (81 percent) believe that health care costs have gotten worse over the past five years.[15] Forty-two percent of the HCS respondents indicated that they were not confident in their ability to afford health care in the next ten years without suffering financial hardship. Consumers' cost-sensitivity was also evident in the AHCPR/Kaiser survey, in which 47 percent of the respondents said cost was the primary reason for their decision to change health

plans. Rising insurance copayments and deductibles are caus-
ing consumers to assume more personal responsibility for
direct health care costs. Thus, the ratio of product quality to
price will likely become an increasingly important provider
attribute for the public.

Provider Demographics

Consumer choices are also influenced by demographic and
geographic characteristics. For example, the elderly person is
more apt to respond favorably to a provider that offers chronic
care services, whereas the younger consumer may judge
providers based on convenience and responsiveness. A number
of consumer characteristics (for example, age, sex, education,
income, ethnicity, geographic location, and so on) strongly
influence purchasing decisions and must be considered when
designing report cards targeted for distribution to a particular
market segment.[16]

Information to Include in Provider Report Cards

Consumer demand for information that can be used to evaluate provider quality is growing. More than half of the 1,011
American households that participated in the December 1996
national poll commissioned by the National Coalition on
Health Care said they would like to be better informed about
how to evaluate quality of medical care.[17] In response to this
and other surveys, the President's Advisory Commission on
Consumer Protection and Quality in the Health Care Industry recommended that health care professionals and facilities
provide quality-related information to the public. According
to the commission, some of these data (figure 1-1) should be
routinely provided and other data should be made available
upon request.[18]

Figure 1-1. Performance Measures Recommended by the President's Advisory Commission on Consumer Protection and Quality in the Health Care Industry

Health Professional Information

Routinely provided information:

- Ownership or affiliation agreements with a provider group or institution that would make referral to a particular specialist or facility more likely
- How the provider is compensated

Information to be made available on request:

- Education, board certification, and recertification status
- Years of practice as a physician and as a specialist if so identified
- Consumer satisfaction measures
- Service performance measures
- Corporate form of practice
- Names of hospitals where physicians have admitting privileges
- Experience with performing certain medical or surgical procedures, adjusted for case-mix severity
- Clinical quality performance measures
- Accreditation status (if applicable)
- Availability of translation or interpretation services for non-English-speakers and people with communication disabilities
- Any cancellation, suspension, or exclusion from participation in a federal program or sanction from a federal agency; any suspension or revocation of medical licensure, federal controlled substance license, or hospital privileges

Health Care Facility Information

Routinely provided information:

- Corporate form of the facility
- Accreditation status
- Specialty programs' compliance with established guidelines
- Volume of certain procedures performed
- Consumer satisfaction measures
- Clinical quality measures
- Service performance measures
- Complaint process
- Availability of translation or interpretation services
- Number and credentials of providers of direct patient care
- Affiliation that would make it more likely that referrals would be made within a provider network
- Whether facility has been excluded from any federal health program

Performance Measures

The performance measures viewed as important by the providers themselves and those associated with the health care industry may not be the same ones that consumers find useful. In the AHCPR/Kaiser consumer survey, respondents rated satisfaction data from previous patients as a very influential source in their choice of health plans, physicians, and hospitals.[19] However, when consumers are asked to define the most important attributes they look for in a health care provider, they don't always rank service satisfaction first on their list.

Illustrated by the recent studies summarized below, consumers appear to want to know about convenience and accessibility, ease of appointment scheduling, length of waiting times, ease of access to emergency services, communication and interpersonal skills of caregivers, and how much patient education is furnished.

- When consumers in Oregon were asked to judge the importance of various health plan performance measures, they viewed patient satisfaction measures as one of the most useful indicators of quality. Other provider-specific measures that ranked high included compassion, communication skills, and respectful listening.[20] Oregon researchers also discovered that consumers find most condition-specific performance measures to be of limited value when making a choice among caregivers. The public reported a general lack of understanding of what the indicator represented; for example, whether the rate of low-birth-weight babies delivered is a good or bad outcome. Condition-specific outcome measures also appeared to be of limited value to consumers unless they had relevance to their individual circumstance (for example, mammography rates for women or well-baby care for new mothers).
- In a study of why Medicare beneficiaries disenroll from HMOs, the Department of Health and Human Services

(DHHS) found the most common causes were as follows: patient complaints were not taken seriously, doctors did not provide care when needed, too much emphasis was placed on holding down costs, patients' personal health worsened while enrolled in the HMO, and there were long waits in the primary care doctor's office.[21]

- The Consumer Information Project, funded by the DHHS, found that consumers generally did not want summary satisfaction ratings for their providers because they did not believe they could interpret this information and felt it might be biased. These study findings suggested that consumers want hard data, such as the actual number of days they had to wait for a physician's appointment or how much time patients spent in the physician's waiting room.[22]

Data on Clinical Outcomes

There is considerable debate as to whether data on clinical outcomes should be included on publicly distributed provider-specific report cards. Aside from the challenges of accurately measuring patient outcomes, there is controversy as to which outcomes are most important to patients. Clinicians and patients tend to define "good outcome" differently. For example, surgeons may be concerned about the patient's wound healing and restoration of normal clinical lab values. However, postoperatively, patients are often more interested in their pain, distress, fatigue, and ability to carry out normal life functions. Although caregivers tend to measure patient outcomes based on the degree of improvement in clinical status, patients are more apt to define a good outcome as one that meets their pretreatment expectations (for example, they returned to normal activity levels as quickly as they thought they would; they experienced less pain than anticipated).[23]

However, despite this, satisfaction levels are not necessarily influenced by the patient's achievement or nonachievement of expected outcomes. Kane, Maciejewski, and Finch found that change in patients' clinical or functional status did not appear to influence their evaluation ratings of providers. When judging their satisfaction with care they had received, patients were more likely to focus on their present state of health than on the extent of improvement they had enjoyed.[24]

Report Card Data Broken Down into Categories

What data do consumers want to see in health care provider report cards? Based on the findings of the study results presented in this chapter and the work of hundreds of other researchers who have evaluated the same question, consumer-oriented provider report cards should include data in at least the following four categories:

1. Tangibles (physical facilities, equipment, and appearance of clinical and nonclinical personnel)
2. Responsiveness (service availability and promptness)
3. Assurance (knowledge of clinical and nonclinical personnel, as well as their ability to inspire trust and confidence)
4. Interactions (courtesy, friendliness, and empathy shown by the people delivering services and their ability to provide individualized attention and caring)

Examples of performance measures in each of these categories are listed in figure 1-2. It's also important that consumers have a sense of providers' reliability—how consistently they perform in the key attributes considered important to customers. For this reason, provider-specific reports should include past and current performance measurement results.

Consumer Issues That Define Provider Quality

Even providers find that the intricacies of health care structure, process, and outcomes can make the simplest performance measure a bewildering yardstick of quality. The public cannot be expected to evaluate complex clinical and financial data to

Figure 1-2. Performance Measures for Provider-Specific Report Cards Intended for Public Distribution

Tangibles

- The physical facility meets ADA regulations (e.g., wheelchair accessible, sufficient, and clearly marked handicapped parking spaces, etc.)
- The outside appearance of the physical facility shows evidence of regular routine maintenance
- The inside appearance of the physical facility shows evidence that routine housekeeping functions are performed on a regular basis
- The equipment is regularly maintained according to manufacturer's recommendations
- Waiting room space is adequate for the volume of people to be seen
- Parking space is adequate for the volume of people to be seen
- Number of physical facility violations found during state inspections

Responsiveness

- Percent of patients/clients who were satisfied with the ease of getting appointments for visits or tests
- Waiting times for emergency, urgent, and routine care appointments
- Average amount of time the caregiver spends with each patient/client
- Total nursing care hours provided per patient day (hospital)
- Average number of clinic visits scheduled per hour per physician
- Availability of weekend and after-hours health care services
- Percent of patients/clients reporting that they received a timely response to their questions and problems

Assurance

- Percent of caregivers who are specialty/board certified
- Percent of patients/clients who report they were comfortable/very comfortable caring for themselves following the health care intervention
- Rates of health promotion and disease prevention activities (e.g., immunization rates, participation in smoking cessation programs)
- Rates of screening programs for early detection of disease (e.g., mammography, pap smear, prenatal care)
- Rates of compliance with nationally recognized clinical practice guidelines (e.g., the right treatment and ongoing monitoring for patients with chronic diseases)
- Percent of patients/clients reporting that they received care from the right kind of caregiver (e.g., the caregiver's gender, ethnicity, and language meet the patient's preferences)
- Medical and surgical treatment outcome rates (including morbidity/mortality rates, quality of care, functional status, etc.)

Figure 1-2. (Continued)

- Percent of patients/clients reporting satisfaction with pain management interventions
- Number of disciplinary actions (e.g., censure, revocation of license, nonaccreditation, etc.) taken against the provider by state regulatory agencies or accreditation groups
- Number of formal complaints received about the provider by regulatory agencies and/or consumer "watchdogs" (e.g., state health department, medical licensing board, state department of insurance, etc.)

Interactions
- Percent of patients/clients who report satisfaction with their experience of care
- How often testing and treatment choices are explained to patients/clients (as documented in health records)
- How often patients/clients participate in decision making (as documented in health records)
- How often the clinician's documented plan of care reflects patient/client–defined treatment goals
- How often patient/client–defined treatment goals are met
- Percentage of patients/clients who report that they actively participated in decisions concerning their treatment
- How often caregivers offer advice/assistance to help patients/clients avoid illness and stay healthy (as documented in health records)
- Patient/client ratings of staff friendliness, courtesy, respect, dignity, and other interpersonal issues
- Percent of patients/clients reporting that they were able to get their questions answered
- Percent of patients/clients reporting that they had access to educational materials related to their condition
- Percent of patients/clients reporting that they were kept informed of each step of the health care delivery process (inpatient or outpatient services)

assess provider quality. To select the most appropriate measures of provider performance to include in consumer-oriented health care report cards, it is important to understand how the public judges the quality of a health care provider. A recent Press-Ganey study helps to answer this.[25] This research included responses from 1,007,612 hospital patient surveys from December 1995 to November 1996, representing data from 545 hospitals in 44 states. The top ten issues most closely correlated with the likelihood that patients would recommend the hospital to others were:

1. Staff sensitivity to the inconvenience that health problems and hospitalizations can cause
2. Overall cheerfulness of the hospital
3. Staff concern for patients' privacy
4. Amount of attention paid to patients' special or personal needs
5. Degree to which nurses took patients' health problems seriously
6. Technical skill of nurses
7. Nurses' attitudes toward patients' calling them
8. Degree to which the nurses kept patients adequately informed about tests, treatment, and equipment
9. Friendliness of nurses
10. Promptness in responding to the call button

This survey substantiates how important the "caring" side of health care is to the consumer. People are most likely to base decisions about quality on the factors they can personally measure, such as customer service. For this reason, satisfaction as well as other service-related quality measures are likely to remain influential consumer-focused indicators of provider performance for quite some time. Other clinical and financial indicators of performance, including those suggested by the President's Advisory Commission on Consumer Protection and Quality in the Health Care Industry, are likely to play a more important role in consumer decision making once the public better understands how to interpret the information.

Conclusion

Consumers generally do not seek information about health care providers until they or a family member is faced with a health problem, although the trend toward learning more about health provider services is growing. When the time comes to select a provider, most users of health care services tend to rely on the opinion and advice of friends and family, preferring to trust in the experience of people they know. However, other factors do come into play in making that choice, including relying on the opinion of experts, preferring certain provider demographics over others, being attracted by specific provider personal attributes, and, more than ever before, cost.

As public interest in provider information grows, providers are faced with deciding what data need to be included in consumer report cards. Research shows that various performance measures are particularly important to the users of health care, such as wait times, ease of scheduling appointments, convenience, and so on. Although there is interest in information on clinical outcomes, clinical outcomes are less easy to define in a way that both provider and consumer understand. A recent Press-Ganey study provides guidelines for providers on how consumers generally define quality with regard to health care service and reveals that most consumers tend to use factors they can personally measure, such as customer service.

References

1. David B. Nash, "Report on Report Cards," *Health Policy Newsletter* 2, no. 5 (May 1998): 1–2.

2. Uwe Reinhardt, "Measuring Outcomes and Processes Will Lead to Health Care Value for Patients and Consumers," conference presentation, Measures in the Marketplace: Integrating Methods and Information into Health Care (Stratis Health's Quality Watch '97 conference), May 5, 1997.

3. John C. Mowen and Michael Minor, *Consumer Behavior,* 5th ed. (Upper Saddle River, NJ: Prentice Hall, 1998), p. 242.

4. Philip Kotler and Gary Armstrong, *Marketing: An Introduction,* 4th ed. (Upper Saddle River, NJ: Prentice Hall, 1997), p. 217.

5. John C. Mowen and Michael Minor, *Consumer Behavior,* 5th ed. (Upper Saddle River, NJ: Prentice Hall, 1998), pp. 246–47.

6. HealthScope Web site: http://www.healthscope.org/hospital/quality.htm (June 1998).

7. Daniel R. Longo, Garland Land, Wayne Schramm, Judy Fraas, Barbara Hoskins, and Vicky Howell, "Consumer Reports in Health Care: Do They Make a Difference in Patient Care?" *Journal of the American Medical Association* 278, no. 19 (November 19, 1997): 1579–84.

8. V. Dato, L. Ziskin, M. Fulcomer, R. M. Martin, and K. Knoblauch, "Average Postpartum Length of Stay for Uncomplicated Deliveries— New Jersey, 1995," *Morbidity and Mortality Weekly Report* 45, no. 32 (August 1996): 700–704.

9. Sandra Robinson and Mollyann Brodie, "Understanding the Quality Challenge for Health Care Consumers: The Kaiser/AHCPR Survey," *Joint Commission Journal on Quality Improvement* 23, no. 5 (May 1997): 229.

10. SPRY Foundation, *Making Decisions about Long Term Care: Voices of Elderly People and Their Families* (Washington, DC: SPRY Foundation, 1996).

11. Philip Kotler and Gary Armstrong, *Marketing: An Introduction,* 4th ed. (Upper Saddle River, NJ: Prentice Hall, 1997), pp. 37–38.

12. John C. Mowen and Michael Minor, *Consumer Behavior,* 5th ed. (Upper Saddle River, NJ: Prentice Hall, 1998), p. 491.

13. Susan Edgman-Levitan and Paul D. Cleary, "What Information Do Consumers Want and Need?" *Health Affairs* 15, no. 4 (winter 1996): 47–53.

14. Shoshanna Sofaer, "How Will We Know We Got It Right? Aims, Benefits and Risks of Consumer Information Initiatives Survey," *Journal on Quality Improvement* 23, no. 5 (May 1997): 263.

15. Employee Benefits Research Institute, "Health Confidence Survey Finds Americans Satisfied, Mixed Up & Worried" (press release), May 14, 1998.

16. Charles D. Schewe and Reuben M. Smith, *Marketing Concepts and Applications* (New York: McGraw-Hill Book Company, 1980), pp. 134–42.

17. International Communications Research, "How Americans Perceive the Health Care System," national survey conducted for the National Coalition on Health Care, WWW document, January 1997, URL: http://www.nchc.org/perceive.html.

18. Advisory Commission on Consumer Protection and Quality in the Health Care Industry, *Consumer Bill of Rights and Responsibilities,* report to the President of the United States, Washington, DC, November 1997.

19. Agency for Health Care Policy and Research Center for Health Information Dissemination, "AHCPR and Kaiser Examine Consumers' Use of Quality Information," *Research Activities* 12, no. 199 (December 1996): 10–11.

20. Judith H. Hibbard and J. J. Jewett, "Will Quality Report Cards Help Consumers?" *Health Affairs* 16, no. 3 (March 1997): 218–28.

21. Susan Edgman-Levitan and Paul D. Cleary, "What Information Do Consumers Want and Need?" *Health Affairs* 15, no. 4 (winter 1996): 47.

22. J. McGee, S. Shoshanna, and B. Kreling, *Findings from Focus Groups Conducted for the National Committee for Quality Assurance (NCQA) Medicare and Medicaid Consumer Information Project* (Washington, DC: National Committee for Quality Assurance, July 1996).

23. Alain Leplège and Sonia Hunt, "The Problem of Quality of Life in Medicine," *Journal of the American Medical Association* 278, no. 1 (July 2, 1997): 47–50.

24. Robert L. Kane, Matthew Maciejewski, and Michael Finch, "The Relationship of Patient Satisfaction with Care and Clinical Outcomes," *Medical Care* 35, no. 7 (July 1997): 714–30.

25. T. McIntosh, "Empathy: Why Patients Recommend Hospitals," *Healthcare Benchmarks* 4 (1997): 39.

CHAPTER TWO

Communicating the Provider's Message to the Public

Mary M. Krieg, RN,C, MS
Patrice L. Spath, BA, ART

The consumer movement in health care is changing the way providers are doing business, as evidenced by a recent study conducted by Northwestern University's Institute for Health Services Research in conjunction with the accounting firm KPMG.[1] Individual consumers and health care executives in organizations nationwide were surveyed to solicit details regarding the growing impact of consumers in the health care industry. Among other findings, researchers discovered that today's health care consumers are looking for information in a sea of data and are making choices based on what they are discovering about providers and health plans. David Nash, director of the Office of Health Policy Research, Jefferson Medical College, Philadelphia, suggests that central to the consumer movement in health care is the evolution in consumers'"information empowerment."[2] An element of this empowerment is the public's growing desire for useful data they can use to make purchasing choices.

Chapter 1 discussed the attributes that appear to be important to consumers when making provider selections, as well as examples of performance measures that providers can include in their publicly available performance reports. It is quite likely the specific areas on which measures should focus will continue to be refined. The American Medical Accreditation Program[SM] (AMAP[SM]), the Joint Commission on Accreditation of Healthcare Organizations (JCAHO), and the National Committee for Quality Assurance (NCQA) are currently working on a collaborative initiative to develop measurement programs that can help consumers and payers make purchasing decisions.[3] The Foundation for Accountability (FACCT), a not-for-profit organization headquartered in Portland, Oregon, is pilot testing consumer-friendly performance measures for a number of medical conditions.[4] FACCT is also working with several national health care professional organizations and consumer groups to develop methods for disseminating the measurement results to the public.

Even when useful performance data are made available to the general public, consumers don't always appear to be using them to make provider selection decisions. The Pennsylvania Health Care Cost Containment Council has published the *Consumer Guide to Coronary Artery Bypass Graft (CABG) Surgery* since 1992. This report details the CABG surgery risk-adjusted mortality ratings of all cardiac surgeons and hospitals in the state. Schneider and Epstein recently studied the impact of this publication on consumer decision making by examining the use of these data by patients who had undergone surgery at select hospitals in Pennsylvania.[5] They found that only 20 percent of the 474 patients surveyed were aware of the report and even less (12 percent) knew of the report prior to their CABG surgery. The study authors conclude that further efforts aimed at developing quality information for general audiences should explore the use of Internet-based and other media for communicating report card data. It is apparent that although debates about the appropriateness of various measures of health care performance continue, providers should also be examining the effectiveness of various methods for disseminating these data to the public.

This chapter describes the decision steps involved in developing a provider report card and various distribution strategies. These recommendations outline a reasonable framework for report card development that all direct-care health organizations can use in designing and disseminating performance data to the public.

Decision Steps in Designing a Provider Report Card

The message a provider organization communicates to the public is influenced by its vision (what it wishes to be known for), its mission (how the organization plans to achieve its vision), and its quality definition (the organization's quality priorities). Together, these should provide a focus for the key attributes of organizational performance that will be included on its report card.

Step 1. Define the Purpose of the Report Card

This step involves determining the target audience (for example, previous patients, the community-at-large, potential markets you want to enter, decision makers, and subcategories or segmented populations of the current market) and defining the purpose of the report (for example, what you want the recipients to learn and what actions you expect them to take after reviewing the data). A clear statement of purpose will make the selection of performance measures and the data presentation style much easier.

Step 2. Determine Performance Measures

Considering the purpose the provider has defined for its report card, the provider should then determine which performance measures will best serve this purpose. Numerous examples of performance measures that might be appropriate for a publicly available performance report are listed in chapter 1.

An important consideration is whether to include comparative data from other facilities in the report card. Some consumers apparently want comparative data to help them make choices among providers. For example, researchers in the Consumer Information Project found that consumers wanted to know how their providers compare with national norms.[6] Consumers also requested data showing comparisons relevant to their age, sex, and health status. The public's desire for comparative data has emerged in other consumer studies.[7] For example, in the recent examination of patients' use of the Pennsylvania Health Care Cost Containment Council's *Consumer Guide to Coronary Artery Bypass Graft (CABG) Surgery,* a number of patients expressed interest in comparative data on mortality outcomes and claimed they would use such reports in their decision making.[8]

However, whether comparative data can be accurately interpreted by the public is a lingering question that has yet to be answered. In a study conducted by McGee and Knutson for the Minnesota Department of Employee Relations, researchers found that the impact of comparative information on employees' choice of a health plan depended largely on how they interpreted the information and whether the results differed from their expectations.[9] Interviews with employees revealed that data interpretations were highly personal and that people tended to draw different conclusions from the same information.

In determining the content of the report card, the provider organization should consider the effect of the purpose of the report and the availability of data.

Purpose The purpose of the report card should drive its content. If one of the goals of disseminating performance data is to demonstrate the efficiency of the organization and its practitioners, the report card should illustrate proper utilization of resources, efficacy of services, and sound financial management. Utilization data for a hospital could include average length of stay (ALOS) for all discharges and particular diseases and conditions, average cost per discharge, and average cost for selected procedures, tests, or studies.

Financial management data can also be used to show that the organization functions in a cost–effective manner. Some indicators of financial management include operating margins, ratio of current assets to current liabilities, age of accounts receivable, and the like. For example, Community-General Hospital in Syracuse, New York, wishes to show consumers that it is a cost-efficient facility. For this reason, one portion of its publicly available report card includes financial indicators. (See figure 2-1.) To allow consumers the ability to compare Community-General's performance with that of other hospitals in New York, comparative statistics from the Central New York Health Systems Agency Financial Ratio report are also provided.

If one of the goals of the provider report card is to demonstrate high-quality patient care, measures of safety can be included in the performance report (such as annual number of patient falls and medication errors, surgical wound and other nosocomial infection rates, complication rates, and so on). Clinical quality and appropriateness of care are other major areas of concern to consumers. These attributes can be demonstrated by reporting various measures, such as mortality, morbidity, disposition, readmission rates, mobility at discharge versus admission, cesarean section and vaginal birth after c-section (VBAC) rates, hysterectomy rates, average "door-to-drug" administration time for patients receiving thrombolysis, number of diabetic patients receiving an annual eye exam, and childhood immunization rates. A drawback to reporting these measures is that the average person may not understand the significance of the data they are being asked to interpret. This is why appropriateness and outcome data in a report card should be accompanied by explanations, such as those provided by Group Health Cooperative (Seattle, Washington) in the multipage performance measurement report they publish for consumers. Figure 2-2 shows an excerpt from the

Figure 2-1. Financial Indicators from the Community-General Hospital Quality Report Card

		CNYHSA[b]	
SELECTED FINANCIAL INDICATORS **1992[a]**			
	CGH	**Median**	**Favorable** **Direction**
Operating margin ratio	0.021	.001	Above median
Current ratio	1.83	1.40	Above median
Accounts receivable age (days)	72.12	79.01	Below median
Cash flow to debt	0.30	0.10	Above median
Average age of facility (years)	7.64	9.97	Below median

[a]*1992 is the most recent year for which comparison information is available from the CNYHSA.*
[b]*Source: Central New York Health Systems Agency Financial Ratio Report (February 22, 1994)*

Observation:
Community-General Hospital's financial performance is better than comparison levels.

Reprinted, with permission, from Community-General Hospital, Syracuse, New York.

maternity care section of the 1996 report. As illustrated, the report includes prenatal care rates for patients seen by Group Health Cooperative physicians, comparative data from the NCQA Quality Compass report, the performance goal established by the *Healthy People 2000* initiative, and a brief explanation of the importance of early prenatal care.

If an organization wishes to demonstrate to the public that former patients are happy with the care they received, patient satisfaction data should be a cornerstone of its report card. (See chapter 6 for a discussion of patient satisfaction measures.) The Cleveland Health Quality Choice Coalition's report (figure 2-3) is an excellent example of how to share satisfaction data

Figure 2-2. Group Health Cooperative's Effectiveness of Care Report—Maternity Care: Prenatal Care in the First Trimester

	1996
Women with live births during the reporting period, sample population	411
Women with live births during the reporting period who had a prenatal care visit in their first trimester	345
Prenatal care rate	83.9%

Background

Early prenatal screening identifies high-risk women, resulting in appropriate intervention and treatment.

Measure

The rate of women experiencing a live birth during the reporting year who had a prenatal care visit 26 to 44 weeks prior to delivery

Improvement

Group Health emphasizes education as a key aspect of entry into prenatal care. Typically, the first prenatal visit is an educational session, an encounter not captured by this measure. This educational session assures that women have immediate information on topics such as nutrition, exercise, and use of medications and other substances at the earliest possible time. The session answers questions about prenatal testing, addresses risk factors in pregnancy, and provides resources on potential problems to watch for in the early weeks of pregnancy. Group Health uses a variety of models for this session, including classes, one-to-one sessions with an "Early Pregnancy Advisor" (an RN), and joint nurse/physician office visits.

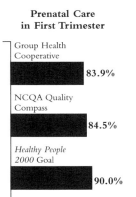

Prenatal Care in First Trimester

Group Health Cooperative: 83.9%

NCQA Quality Compass: 84.5%

Healthy People 2000 Goal: 90.0%

Figure 2-3. Excerpt from Cleveland Health Quality Choice Report on Hospital Performance

CLEVELAND HEALTH QUALITY CHOICE • NOVEMBER 11, 1997 SUMMARY REPORT

CHART 1A
Hospital Patient Satisfaction/Medical & Surgical

Global Satisfaction

(Composite score of three questions asking if patient would return, brag about the hospital to others, or recommend it to friends and family.)

	Report 6 10/94–3/95	Report 7 4/95–9/95	Report 8 10/95–3/96	Report 9 4/96–9/96	Report 10 10/96–3/97
Allen Memorial	↔	↔	↔	↔	↔
Cleveland Clinic	▲	▲	▲	▲	▲
Columbia St. John West Shore	▼	▼	↔	↔	↔
Columbia St. Luke's Med Ctr	↔	↔	↔	⇩	↔
Columbia St. Vincent Charity	↔	↔	↔	↔	↔
Community Health Partners	↔	↔	↔	⇩	▼
EMH Regional Med Ctr	↔	▲	⇧	▲	↔
Fairview	↔	↔	⇩	▼	↔
Lake East	↔	↔	↔	↔	↔
Lake West	▼	↔	↔	↔	↔
Lakewood	⇧	↔	↔	⇧	↔
Lutheran	↔	⇧	↔	↔	↔
Marymount	↔	↔	↔	↔	↔
Meridia Euclid	↔	⇧	↔	↔	↔

This Summary Report includes outcome information for the 11 specific process measures that comprise Total Process Satisfaction (Table 1B). Listed here are results for Report 10 (discharges between October 1, 1996, and March 31, 1997). No data from previous reports are presented for individual process scales.

Housekeeping	Information	Living Arrangements	Nursing Care	Physician Care
⇧	⇔	⬆	⇔	⇔
⇩	⇔	⬇	⇔	⇔
⇔	⇔	⬆	⇔	⇔
⇔	⇔	⇩	⇔	⇔
⇔	⇔	⇔	⇔	⇔
⇔	⬇	⇩	⬇	⇔
⇔	⇔	⇧	⇔	⇔
⇔	⇔	⬇	⇔	⇔
⬆	⇧	⇔	⇧	⇔
⬆	⇧	⬆	⬆	⇩
⇔	⇔	⇔	⇔	⇔
⇔	⇔	⇔	⇔	⇔
⇔	⇔	⇔	⇔	⬇
⇔	⇔	⇔	⇧	⇔

How to Interpret the Symbols

⬆ Patient satisfaction <u>higher than predicted.</u> There is only a 1 in 100 chance that this hospital is listed in this group by chance alone.

⇧ Patient satisfaction <u>higher than predicted.</u> There is only a 1 in 20 chance that this hospital is listed in this group by chance alone.

⇔ Patient satisfaction <u>as predicted.</u>

⇩ Patient satisfaction <u>lower than predicted.</u> There is only a 1 in 20 chance that this hospital is listed in this group by chance alone.

⬇ Patient satisfaction <u>lower than predicted.</u> There is a 1 in 100 chance that this hospital is listed in this group by chance alone.

NOTES TO CHART 1C

• Data gathered using the Patient Viewpoint® Survey.

• Satisfaction of hospitals compared to their own outcome range and grouped by statistical comparison to Cleveland area. Questionnaires sent to 600 patients at each hospital asking about 11 areas of hospital service.

with the public. Using a *Consumer Reports* type of graphic format, global satisfaction data as well as satisfaction with specific attributes (housekeeping, information, living arrangements, nursing care, and physician care) are displayed. Consumers can also see trends in patient satisfaction results.

Availability of Data   The most common measures found on provider report cards are those that can be easily gathered from administrative or claims data showing volume statistics (for example, number of clients treated in various disease categories, number of clients served, and so on), mortality and complication rates, length of treatment (for example, hospital ALOS, number of clinic visits or home care visits per episode of care, and so on), hospital readmission rates, cesarean section and VBAC rates, and charges (e.g., average hospital stay charges, average clinic visit charges, and total charges for an episode of care).

In many instances, the data necessary to fulfill the purpose of the provider report may not be readily accessible in existing databases. In such situations, organizations have two choices. They can either limit report card measures to available data elements and potentially compromise their primary objectives in sharing data with the public, or they can develop new data sources. Organizations may find they need to gather additional clinical data elements from patient records and conduct patient telephone surveys to fulfill the goal of reporting detailed patient satisfaction and clinical outcome data to consumers.

Step 3. Make the Report Card Accessible to Users

Public-oriented, provider-specific report cards must be presented in a manner the public can understand. Even if the report card includes data about key attributes that are important to customers, the public is likely to disregard the information if it is not properly packaged or readable.

Packaging   Packaging involves the various elements that make the content of the report understandable and accessible. As the following examples show, the organization of the information, the inclusion of clear graphics, and conciseness will make the card easy for readers to use:

- One group involved in designing and disseminating a health plan report card is the Oregon Consumer Scorecard Consortium.[10] The purpose of this scorecard initiative is to aid consumers in choosing a health plan. The project focused primarily on design of a scorecard that could be used by Medicaid clients, although the study results have implications for all consumer-oriented health care report cards. The focus group meetings that were held with Medicaid recipients throughout Oregon revealed an important issue relevant to report card design, which is that the amount of data presented on report cards should be limited in number to keep from overwhelming consumers' ability to assimilate the information.
- The performance report of Mercy Hospital Medical Center, Des Moines, Iowa, is a good example of a consumer-friendly hospital report card. (See figure 2-4.) The general public can easily understand the brief explanations, and colorful graphics are used to display inpatient and outpatient quality indicators. This report is distributed in printed form, and an abbreviated version is available on Mercy Hospital's Web site at: http://www.mercydesmoines.org.
- Another good example of a concise provider report is the one recently released by the California Office of Statewide Health Planning and Development (OSHPD). The OSHPD's latest report studied outcomes of heart attack patients within 30 days of admission at more than 400 hospitals statewide between 1991 and 1993. Although the report is not without critics, it does represent the data in such a manner as to allow a quick analysis. With only a few page

Figure 2-4. Mercy Hospital Medical Center Quality Report Card

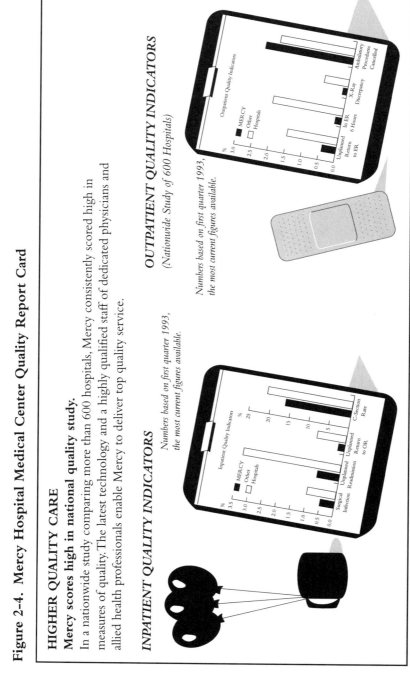

HIGHER QUALITY CARE

Mercy scores high in national quality study.

In a nationwide study comparing more than 600 hospitals, Mercy consistently scored high in measures of quality. The latest technology and a highly qualified staff of dedicated physicians and allied health professionals enable Mercy to deliver top quality service.

INPATIENT QUALITY INDICATORS

Numbers based on first quarter 1993, the most current figures available.

OUTPATIENT QUALITY INDICATORS

(Nationwide Study of 600 Hospitals)

Numbers based on first quarter 1993, the most current figures available.

Reprinted, with permission, from Mercy Hospital Medical Center.

flips, a fairly intelligent layperson can determine which of the state's hospitals are best and worst at treating heart attack victims based on outcomes. An abbreviated version of this report is available on the Healthscope Web site at: http://www.healthscope.org/hospital/h_attack/index.htm.

- The Center for Quality of Care Research and Education at the Harvard School of Public Health suggests that clinical performance measures can be useful information for consumers if they are presented in an understandable format and with accompanying text about the care that is recommended by practice guidelines and the outcomes that can be expected for each condition.[11] For example, if the hospital chooses to report the "percentage of new mothers who were breastfeeding their newborn baby at the time of discharge," this information could be accompanied by a statement such as "breastfeeding, even for a short period, has many health benefits for babies."[12]

- FACCT is working to create a consumer information framework that is intended to provide measurement data to the public in a manner that allows for quality comparisons among health care providers.[13] The communication framework, which will continue to be tested and refined through 1999, organizes quality information into five areas: (1) delivering the basics of good care (skill, communication, coordination of care); (2) keeping people healthy; (3) helping people get better when they get sick; (4) assisting the chronically ill to cope with illness; and (5) adapting to the needs of patients and their families when health needs or functional abilities change dramatically.

Readability   It is important to consider the readability of the performance report given the provider's intended audience. Too often communications produced by health care organizations baffle the public because the authors don't take into account their audience's literacy levels, reading skills, and thinking style.[14] A 1992 survey by the U.S. Department of

Education's National Center for Education Statistics estimated that about 21 percent of the American population over the age of 16 have only rudimentary reading and writing skills.[15] Before creating printed materials for distribution to its target audience, the provider should find out more about its audience's literacy levels. Adult literary estimates for various geographic areas in the United States can be obtained at the Web site of the Comprehensive Adult Student Assessment System (http://www.casas.org/). Then readability tests should be conducted to determine the reading level of the materials before they are disseminated to the target audience. Readability also relates to the layout and graphic design of printed materials. If the data are not presented in a visually appealing, easy-to-read manner, the chances of retaining the attention of the intended audience are significantly reduced.

Writing about health care services often requires the use of some technical language. However, the way the message is presented (writing style, vocabulary, typography, layout, graphics, and color) can favorably affect whether it is read and understood.[16] Other factors to consider when creating report cards that will be accepted by the public include the following:

- Messages must clearly convey information to ensure the public's understanding and to limit the chances for misunderstanding or inappropriate action. As much as possible, jargon, technical terms or phrases, abbreviations, and acronyms should be avoided.
- The main points should be stressed, repeated, and never hidden within less strategically important information.
- Graphics should be simple and uncluttered and used to reinforce, not compete, with the text.
- The tone of the message should be truthful, honest, and as complete as possible.
- The spokesperson and source of the information should be credible and trustworthy.
- The special needs of ethnic minorities (language, varying needs, values, and beliefs) should be considered.

Before final production, pretest your report card with the target audience(s) to ensure that they understand your message and that you've achieved the stated purpose of your report card initiative (for example, to convey new facts, alter attitudes, or change purchasing behavior).

Dissemination Strategies

A number of methods may be used to convey performance data to the public. These vary greatly in scope, cost, level of sophistication, and number of people reached. Most organizations already producing publicly available performance data use a variety of dissemination strategies. Following are some examples:

- The first report of the Minnesota Health Data Institute (MHDI) about the quality of the state's health plans was distributed to the public in three formats.[17] Several newspapers published about a million copies of the 12-page insert entitled, "You and Your Health Plan: A Minnesota Survey." The report was formatted for the Internet and made available through MHDI's corporate Web page. MHDI also published an executive report geared toward policy makers and individuals interested in health care reform. As in Minnesota, the process of dissemination of most report card data relies primarily on media such as television and newspapers. An increasing number of performance reports are also available on provider Internet Web sites.
- The Oregon Consumer Scorecard Consortium found that consumers wanted health plan performance data in several formats.[18] Although the focus groups believed that multiple media presentations (computer kiosks, videos, and telephone backup) were useful, they agreed that written information should always be available. Consumers also thought it would be helpful to have access to a live person (by phone) to answer questions consumers may have about the data.

Dissemination tactics can be divided into two major groups—personal methods and impersonal methods. Performance measurement can be distributed in person by facility representatives during public events (for example, wellness conventions, talks to service organizations, telemarketing, and so on). However, data can also be distributed through impersonal channels, such as newsletters, newspapers, press releases, and yellow page advertisements, and over the Internet. When considering distribution choices, the provider should keep in mind the stated purpose of its report card initiative and the amount of resources it is willing to expend. It's unlikely the provider will recoup its costs by selling the report to the public. When patients in Pennsylvania were asked how much they'd be willing to pay for the *Consumer Guide to Coronary Artery Bypass Graft (CABG) Surgery,* most said they would not pay more than $20 and more than one-third said they expected to obtain the information without charge.[19]

A recent survey of the public's use of quality data on health plans revealed that consumers rely heavily on their physician's recommendations when it comes to choosing a health plan or a hospital.[20] Pennsylvania researchers also concurred that physicians are a very important source of information for patients about the quality of cardiac surgeons.[21] For this reason, report card dissemination strategies should include initiatives designed to educate caregivers about the report and how to use it in discussions with patients. The Florida Hospital Association is doing just that. This association has developed two pamphlets, "The Physician's Guide to the Hospital Performance Reports" (figure 2-5) and "The Nurses Guide to the Hospital Performance Reports," which describe the document published by the Florida Agency for Health Care Administration (AHCA). Not only do these pamphlets explain the data and the methodology used by the Florida AHCA to create the report, but there is also a brief discussion of how to help patients use the guide. Patient-caregiver partnerships designed

Figure 2-5. The Physician's Guide to the Florida Hospital Performance Reports

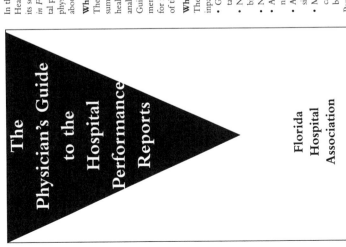

The Physician's Guide to the Hospital Performance Reports

Florida Hospital Association

In the next couple of weeks, the Florida Agency for Health Care Administration (AHCA) is expected to release its second report on hospitals, the *1997 Guide to Hospitals in Florida*, which uses 1995 billing data to examine hospital performance. This document should help you, the physician, answer any questions your patients may ask about the report.

Why was the Guide to Hospitals in Florida created?

The initial purpose for the Guide was to provide consumers with information so they can make "informed" health care decisions. However, as AHCA proceeded to analyze the data, it realized that the primary users of the Guide would be hospitals for their internal quality assessment activities, using the Guide to identify opportunities for improvement. AHCA will release a consumer version of the Guide at a later date.

What is included in the report?

The Guide includes the following information on hospital inpatient services only. The Guide shows:

- General hospital information (ownership, beds, accreditation status)
- Number of deliveries, cesarean rate, and VBAC (vaginal birth after c-section)
- Number of discharges for each of the 16 service lines
- Average charges (observed, expected, and statistical significance)
- Average length of stay (observed, expected, and statistical significance)
- Mortality rate (observed, expected, and statistical significance only for selected service lines—see those noted below)

Performance data are shown for the following services:

Cardiology	Cardiac surgery
Pulmonary medicine	Gastroenterology
Medical oncology*	Neurology
Neurosurgery*	Other medicine
General surgery*	Orthopedics*
Obstetrics*	Gynecology*
Urology*	Pediatrics*
Neonatology*	Vascular and thoracic surgery**

*Mortality rates will not be reported for these services

**New service line for the 1997 Guide

How are the data adjusted?

To determine the "expected" values for each hospital, the average performance of groups of similar patients was calculated, adjusting for the following: severity of illness, race, socioeconomic status, payer, age, sex, whether the patient was terminal, and whether or not the patient was transferred in, and whether or not the patient was terminal. In addition, patient volume, teaching status, trauma center, percentage of patients transferred in, percentage of indigent patients, and geographic input prices were included as hospital adjustment factors. Outliers (patients who are significantly different from other patients), patients leaving against medical advice, and patients transferred to another hospital were excluded from the analysis. Charges and length of stay (LOS) outliers are excluded from the charges and LOS analysis but not from the mortality analysis.

AHCA uses one of the best severity adjustment systems available; however, none of the current systems completely account for patient differences. Caution must be exercised in ascribing significance to any individual value derived. They should be considered as only a few of many indicators of the actual performance of a hospital. While

(Continued on next page)

Figure 2-5. (Continued)

the additional "risk adjustment" method created by University of Florida researchers improves the analysis, this analysis is not perfect.

What do the numbers mean?

The data show how a hospital performed *compared to what was expected*, given a similar mix of patients. The expected values were derived using the quarterly patient data reported by all of Florida's acute care hospitals to AHCA. For a particular hospital, direct comparisons can be made in looking at each service line for these variables:

Observed value shows actual experience of the hospital

Expected value shows what the average performance of the "typical" Florida hospital would be given a similar mix of patients

The following symbols characterize how each hospital compares to others in the same service line, in terms of observed vs. expected performance:

- Indicates the 15% of hospitals with the most favorable performance on this measure (statistically significant, $p < .05$)

o Indicates hospitals whose performance differs significantly from other hospitals but not enough to place them in the top or bottom 15% of hospitals

■ Indicates the 15% of hospitals with the least favorable performance on this measure (statistically significant, $p < .05$)

– Indicates that there is no statistically significant difference. In other words, the minus sign, "-," does not indicate a negative performance.

Thus, the key information is how a particular hospital performed compared to what was "expected" of that hospital, given its mix of patients and its other characteristics. *Direct comparisons between hospitals will lead to misinterpretation of the data because the patient populations vary.* Thus, comparing data for several hospitals will lead to misinterpretation of the data. *Consumers are urged to consult their physician and other health care professionals before using the data for their health care decisions.*

What has changed from the 1996 Report?

The format will stay the same as last year but there are some important changes to the way the numbers are calculated. Two changes affecting the risk adjustment methodology are factors for whether or not the hospital is a trauma center and for the percentage of patients age 75 years and older. These adjustments were added to the 1997 report to better characterize the patient population each hospital serves. Trauma patients and the age of a patient also impact the severity and resources required to treat a patient.

Two changes were made to the actual data. First, hospitals were allowed to identify which patients were terminal or under hospice care. These patients were excluded from the analysis for mortality rates. Second, some of the service line definitions were modified based on discussions with physician specialty groups.

Can you compare the information to 1996?

No. As mentioned above, the model used to calculate the expected values is slightly different. Thus, hospital performance in the 1997 Guide cannot be compared to the 1996 Guide.

Additionally, hospitals had found problems with their data and resubmitted the corrected information to AHCA for the 1996 report. For example, some of the hospitals were not reporting all the conditions affecting patients. Because the patient severity is determined by *all* the conditions affecting the patient, some hospitals had patient populations that appeared to be less severe than they actually were.

How can I help my patients use the Guide?

Since the Guides are not necessarily "consumer-friendly," you can help your patients by educating them on what the data mean and how the guides can be used. Explain to them that these scores are not quality indicators. Even though charges are used in the report, this does not reflect what a patient will actually pay. What is actually paid is dependent upon the contract negotiated between the patient's insurance carrier and the hospital.

Mortality is also a difficult indicator to understand, since death is a rare occurrence in the hospital. Overall, only 3% of the 1.7 million patients treated in the hospital die each year.

What does it say about my practice?

This report shows only aggregate data on hospitals. Physician-specific data or information on physician practice styles is not included in this report. While there has been some discussion about looking at individual physicians, as in New York and Pennsylvania, the state has not yet proceeded forward on it.

FHA staff resources: Kim Streit or Susie White
407/841-6230

Reprinted, with permission, from the Florida Hospital Association.

to enhance the public's understanding and use of provider report cards should be an important component of the dissemination process.

The design and public dissemination of provider-specific report cards requires that many strategic decisions be jointly made by administrative and physician leaders. Efforts are already under way by many different organizations. The products of the labors of these "pioneers" should serve as a starting point for determining how your organization wishes to approach the topic of public-oriented report cards. The significant issues related to taking your performance message to the public are summarized in figure 2-6. Use this checklist to ensure that all important elements are addressed by your organization.

Figure 2-6. Checklist of Report Card Design and Dissemination Considerations

- ☑ The organization has clearly defined vision, mission, and quality definition statements.
- ☑ Performance measures that support the vision, mission, and quality definition of the organization have been selected.
- ☑ The target audience(s) for the public-oriented report card has been identified.
- ☑ The purpose of the public-oriented report card has been clearly defined.
- ☑ If comparative data from other similar facilities are available, a decision has been made as to whether these data will be included on the report card for all measures or only selected measures.
- ☑ Feasible report card distribution methods have been selected.
- ☑ Distribution channels chosen for the report card are credible and will ensure the information reaches the target audience(s).
- ☑ The literacy level of the targeted audience(s) has been considered in the writing and design of report card materials.
- ☑ The special needs of ethnic minority populations have been considered in the writing and design of the report card materials.
- ☑ The layout and graphic design of the report card enhance readability.
- ☑ The final version of the report card is pretested with the target audience(s) before distribution.
- ☑ Tactics for educating caregivers in how to use the report card in discussions with patients have been developed.

Conclusion

If provider-specific performance data are expected to influence the health care consumer's decision-making process, providers must break through the "information clutter" of today's society. The data contained in provider report cards should be based on what the target audience perceives as most important and what it wants to know. If the reports only contain what providers think is most important or interesting, it's unlikely the public will take notice of their message.

Despite the controversy and uncertainty of what to include in provider-specific report cards, a number of organizations are already creating and distributing performance measurement data reports to the public. Many have developed "scorecards" that contain clinical quality, cost-effectiveness, and service satisfaction data. The quest for the "perfect" report card should not preclude organizations from attending to the important related consideration—consumer education.

Providers must take a leading role in educating consumers in the availability and use of performance measurement data. Studies of current report card efforts suggest that few providers discuss performance measurement data with their patients. Yet people view their personal caregiver as one of the more credible sources of information about the quality of providers and health plans. Caregivers must assume a leadership position in shaping the public's health care quality expectations. If providers do not address this educational role, insurers, the government, or the public media will be the ones interpreting comparative information for the users of health care.

References

1. KPMG Peat Marwick LLP, *New Voices: Consumerism in Health Care*, executive summary of telephone research study conducted in 1997 (Atlanta, GA: KPMG, 1998).

2. David B. Nash, "From the Editor: Consumerism in Health Care," *Health Policy Newsletter* 11, no. 3 (September 1998): 1–2.

3. Joint Commission on Accreditation of Healthcare Organizations, "Nation's Three Leading Health Care Quality Oversight Bodies to Coordinate Measurement Activities," JCAHO press release, WWW document, May 1998, http://www.jcaho.org/news/nb137.htm.

4. Foundation for Accountability, "The FACCT Consumer Information Framework: Bringing Consumers Quality Information They Can Use," *Accountability Action* 2, no. 1 (fall 1997): 5–7.

5. Eric C. Schneider and Arnold M. Epstein, "Use of Public Performance Reports: A Survey of Patients Undergoing Cardiac Surgery," *Journal of the American Medical Association* 279, no. 20 (May 27, 1998): 1638–42.

6. Susan Edgman-Levitan and Paul D. Cleary, "What Information Do Consumers Want and Need?" *Health Affairs* 15, no. 4 (winter 1996): 48–49.

7. Research Triangle Institute, *Information Needs for Consumer Choice, Case Study Report,* prepared for the Office of Research and Demonstrations, Health Care Financing Administration (Research Triangle Park, North Carolina, 1995).

8. Eric C. Schneider and Arnold M. Epstein, "Use of Public Performance Reports: A Survey of Patients Undergoing Cardiac Surgery," *Journal of the American Medical Association* 279, no. 20 (May 27, 1998): 1638–42.

9. Jeanne McGee and David Knutson, "Health Care Report Cards: What About Consumers' Perspectives?" *Journal of Ambulatory Care Management* 17, no. 4 (April 1994): 12.

10. Oregon Consumer Scorecard Consortium, *Oregon Consumer Scorecard Project,* NTIS publication no. PB97-117758 (Springfield, VA: National Technical Information Service, 1997).

11. Center for Quality of Care Research and Education, *CONQUEST 1.0: A Computerized Needs-Oriented Quality Measurement Evaluation System,* final report (Rockville, MD: Department of Health and Human Services, Public Health Service, Agency for Health Care Policy and Research, 1996), p. 14.

12. Patrice L. Spath. "Taking the Message Public," in *1998 Medical Quality Management Sourcebook,* J. Mangano, ed. (New York: Faulkner & Gray, 1997), p. 495.

13. Foundation for Accountability, "The FACCT Consumer Information Framework: Bringing Consumers Quality Information They Can Use," *Accountability Action* 2, no. 1 (fall 1997): 5–7.

14. Mark Hochhauser, "Can Your HMO's Documents Pass the Readability Test?" *Managed Care* 16, no. 9 (September 1997): 60A–C.

15. National Center for Education Statistics, *120 Years of American Education: A Statistical Portrait* (Washington, DC: National Center for Education Statistics, 1993).

16. Harold C. McGraw, *Making Health Communications Programs Work: A Planner's Guide,* publication no. 92-1493 (Washington, DC: U.S. Department of Health and Human Services, Public Health Service and National Institutes of Health, April 1992), p. 79.

17. Aileen Kantor, "Consumers: Asking New Questions," *Business & Health* 13, no. 12, Supplement E (1995): 23–29.

18. Oregon Consumer Scorecard Consortium, *Oregon Consumer Scorecard Project,* NTIS publication no. PB97-117758 (Springfield, VA: National Technical Information Service, 1997).

19. Eric C. Schneider and Arnold M. Epstein, "Use of Public Performance Reports: A Survey of Patients Undergoing Cardiac Surgery," *Journal of the American Medical Association* 279, no. 20 (May 27, 1998): 1638–42.

20. Sandra Robinson and Mollyann Brodie, "Understanding the Quality Challenge for Health Consumers: The Kaiser/AHCPR Survey," *Joint Commission Journal on Quality Improvement* 23, no. 5 (1997): 239–44.

21. Eric C. Schneider and Arnold M. Epstein, "Use of Public Performance Reports: A Survey of Patients Undergoing Cardiac Surgery," *Journal of the American Medical Association* 279, no. 20 (May 27, 1998): 1638–42.

CHAPTER THREE

Disseminating Provider Report Cards via the Internet

Charles E. Swain

Creating a provider report card can be difficult. Getting it into the hands of consumers is an even greater challenge. The Oregon Consumer Scorecard Consortium, a state group involved in designing a health plan report, found that successful dissemination of performance measurement data requires a variety of presentation formats and media.[1] Consumer focus groups, sponsored by the Oregon consortium, recommended that multiple reporting options from which consumers could choose would maximize the utility of the available comparative information. Other studies that have looked at methods for distributing quality-of-care data have encouraged a variety of communication methods, including print, television, radio, videotaped presentations, and on-line services.[2]

This chapter addresses how to present provider information to the public via the Internet in an easily accessible and understandable manner. It also includes a brief overview of the resources that will be necessary when starting from scratch (such as start-up costs for a new Web site) or when adding a report card page to an existing Web site.

Using the Internet to Disseminate Provider Report Cards

One clear choice for distributing provider report card results is the Internet. Internet usage is on the rise. According to an August 1998 *Iconocast* census estimate, someone joins the Internet every 1.75 seconds, the equivalent of 49,317 new Internet users every day.[3] Potentially every home in the world with a telephone line can access the World Wide Web (Web). One reason for this intense growth is the public's increasing demand for information about all things that influence their lives, including health care providers. Information on the Web can be accessed at any time, by anyone, and as often as desired. Health care consumers have already indicated that they want information to be readily available when they are faced with a decision (for example, to choose a health plan, secure needed health care, select a primary care physician, and so on).[4] In addition, messages need to be repeated over a long period because people's retention of quality of care information appears to be slight.[5]

Because of the massive growth of the Internet as a source of information, consumers will rely on it more and more for access to health care–related topics. Leland Kaiser, a health care technologies futurist, recently noted that on-line technology won't go away. "In fact," says Kaiser, "it will get better and become a major conduit for information transfer."[6] The President's Advisory Commission on Consumer Protection and Quality in the Health Care Industry suggested in its 1998 report, *Quality First: Better Health Care for All Americans,* that the Internet be used to disseminate performance measurement data to the public.[7]

Every provider's strategy for disseminating performance measurement data to the public must include an Internet-based distribution plan. Although the Web will not be a provider's only communication link to consumers, the Internet is fast becoming the on-line consumers' vehicle of choice for learning more about a particular topic. An April 1998 survey of 10,000 Web users conducted by the Graphics Visualization and Usability Center at Georgia Tech University revealed that the majority of people (86 percent) indicated they used their Web browser to gather information.

A number of health care organizations already have a Web site. For these facilities, transfer of report card data to a page in their Web site merely requires that format and presentation issues be decided. If the provider does not yet have an Internet presence, designing an Internet-based report card will require more resources and a longer lead time.

Developing an Internet Presence

A variety of issues must be considered when developing a new Web presence for an Internet-based communication strategy. Table 3-1 lists the major technical considerations and estimated costs for each of them. In addition, a number of nontechnical issues must be considered when building a report card, such as the time involved, design, and content.

The size of a Web site and its complexity of design affect how long it takes to develop. A simple site created by someone in the organization with an understanding of Web design software could be completed and on-line in seven to ten days. Hiring a Web developer to do most of the site layout and design will incur an increase in time and costs. However, the time required for building the site can be significantly reduced if the provider delivers a thorough site plan to the Web designer. Moreover, Web design firms may provide a template for creating a site plan.

Those organizations wishing to add their performance report card to an already existing Web site should furnish detailed plans to their Webmaster or Web design firm. The

Table 3-1. New Web Page Development: Technical Considerations and Estimated Costs

Technical Consideration	Explanation	Estimated Cost
Establish a domain name	An Internet-recognizable address, called a domain name, must be chosen. A domain name is a unique name that identifies an Internet server or network location. A network location has two or more parts, separated by periods, as in www.yourorganization.com.	$35 per year
Secure a server to host your Web site	The Web site host is a computer where your electronic medium resides. This computer is known as a "Web server." A Web server is a computer that offers services on the World Wide Web (WWW).	One-time setup costs ranging from $50 to $100 and monthly charges of $50 to $100.
Domain name service	This database allows Web browsers to access Web sites by name rather than by the numerically coded site location.	$100 per year
Web site design	The layout and content of each page on your Web site should be carefully designed to meet the needs of your audience.	$750 to $10,000. This wide price range is influenced by the number of pages you have on your Web site and what features you choose. For do-it-yourself organizations, software packages are available for under $200.
Web site promotion	Register with Internet search engines.	Professional promotion fees range from $100 to $500. Do-it-yourself promotion Web sites are available, such as *www.Register-it.com* and *www.netfit.com*.

expense of adding additional pages can be minimized if every-one knows up front what the pages should look like and what features will be included.

Designing an Internet-Based, Consumer-Oriented Report Card

Similar to the report cards each of us received during the course of our school years, the medical quality report card is a tool that presents important and meaningful information. A well-constructed report card reveals essential information about the quality of a health care system, hospital, or provider group and shows how its performance compares with that of peer groups and other organizations.[8] Publishing provider-oriented report cards on the Internet affords organizations a lot of flexibility in educating consumers about what differentiates health care providers and health plans. Many innovative strategies can be used to captivate and maintain the interest of the reader.

The process of designing a Web-based provider report card is very similar to other marketing activities, although the message (performance data) is packaged in a slightly different manner. The following tips can help guide your organization in communicating its quality message on-line.[9] The designers of provider report cards should do the following:

- Focus on content
- Provide relevant information
- Consider the literacy of the audience
- Consider the other unique needs of the audience
- Tailor the content for the on-line medium
- Avoid complicated graphics or statistics
- Develop strong internal linkages and external Web navigation
- Make the report card fun and interactive
- Offer people a reason to return
- Deliver value-added, focused information

Focus on Content

Much of the information to be disseminated on the provider Web site is already available in marketing brochures, press kits, newsletters, and internal literature. However, the data for the Web-based report card must be carefully selected to meet the needs of an audience the provider may know little about. The following questions should be considered when selecting the performance measurement data to be included on a provider Web site:

- Will the user of the information (current and potential customers) find the information to be valuable?
- Can the content be enlivened through humorous or human-interest illustrations, examples, statistics, and quotes?
- Does the content offer users an opportunity for involvement and participation through easy-to-complete forms, letters, surveys, postings to forums and news groups, on-line chats, or contributions of personal stories?

Provide Relevant Information

Oregon researchers have found that consumers find most condition-specific indicators to be of limited value when making a choice among health plans.[10] The same is true for provider-specific report cards. To be worthwhile, performance measures must be relevant to the individual's circumstances. For example, a diabetic patient might be interested in knowing the rate of hospital readmissions for patients with diabetes, whereas healthy adults might be more concerned about how long they will have to wait in the clinic before being seen by a physician.

The Cleveland Clinic Foundation has created several condition-specific Web pages that include outcome measurement data. For example, on the Cleveland Clinic's Web pages dedicated to the topic of epilepsy, the public is offered information on how to judge high-quality health care (http://www

ccf.org/pc/quality/08-15/08-15.htm). They suggest that consumers consider their personal values and beliefs as well as the doctor's qualifications and the hospital's track record. Consumers are also offered data on the success rates of anterior temporal lobe resection at Cleveland Clinic as compared with the success rates reported at other hospitals and patient satisfaction data. A complete listing of Cleveland Clinic's condition-specific Web pages is posted at the following URL: http://www.ccf.org/pc/quality.

Consider the Literacy of the Audience

Consumers may not be able to understand the information given to them by health care providers.[11] This is a twofold problem. First, the words may be too difficult. Designers should keep in mind that the average American has almost 13 years of education but probably reads at the eighth- or ninth-grade level.[12] Second, medical terminology and words commonly used to describe activities in health care organizations are not generally understood vernacular. The readers of the report card won't be able to gain new knowledge if they can't understand the information that's being presented.

For example, one Web-based report card states in the section labeled "Consumer Guide" that people should ask some relevant questions of a health provider before considering using its services. The guide suggests the consumer ask, "How is top management tied into the quality assurance process?" The intent of this guide is to help the consumer make purchasing decisions. However, it is unlikely that the average person is capable of understanding the relevance of this question. It is even more unlikely that the average person will know how to react to the answer he or she might get from providers.

In contrast, another Web-based report card uses a more familiar approach to help consumers choose a health plan. Using an analogy the general public is likely to understand—how an automobile purchasing decision is made—the health plan quality checklist is carefully worded for the literacy level of the average American. Consumers are offered an excellent description of how much effort is involved in the decision-making process for purchasing an automobile as compared to selecting a health service provider.

Consider Other Distinctive Needs of the Audience

Individuals with disabilities or sensory impairments may have trouble accessing some of the materials on the provider's Web site. They may not be able to see graphics because of visual impairments or listen to audio presentations because of hearing impairments. Some individuals have difficulty navigating sites that are poorly organized with unclear directions because they have learning disabilities or use adaptive technology with their computer to access the Web. It is important to follow universal Web page design principles so that all Internet users can get to the information at the Web site regardless of disability or the limitations of their equipment and software.

To see the Web-based report card from the many perspectives of your users, test your Web page with as many Web browsers as you can and always test it with at least one text-based browser. You may want to validate the accessibility of your Web site using the validator program found at the Web site of the Center for Applied Special Technology at http://www.cast.org/bobby/. This program performs a diagnostic on your pages and points out parts that could be inaccessible. Other resources about accessible Web page design are listed in table 3-2.

Tailor the Content for the On-Line Medium

Publishing information on-line is different from creating a marketing brochure. Avoid taking print material and putting it directly on-line. Experience has shown that people who use Web browsers don't want to scroll a document that is more than

**Table 3–2. Sources of Information for Designing Accessible
Web Pages**

Source	Web Site Address
Disabilities, Opportunities, Internetworking and Technology (DO-IT) at the University of Washington includes a list of Internet resources for accessible Web design, as well as other information.	http://weber.u.washington.edu/~doit/
Equal Access to Software and Information's (EASI) Web site provides a good introduction to many issues related to serving patrons with disabilities, including accessible Web design.	http://www.isc.rit.edu/~easi/
The National Center for Accessible Media (NCAM) promotes the use of a Web Access symbol and provides model examples of accessible pages.	http://www.boston.com/wgbh/pages/ncam/currentprojects/webaccess.html
Trace Research and Development Center at the University of Wisconsin-Madison focuses on research and design "to advance the ability of people with disabilities to achieve their life objectives through the use of communication, computer, and information technologies." They include many resources on accessible Web design on their page.	http://www.trace.wisc.edu/

three or four pages. The style needs to be lively, direct, and interesting. The information should provoke thought and entice readers to share their experiences, reactions, and knowledge.

The flexibility of Web page design allows information to be presented in "layers" that provide consumers the opportunity to learn as much or as little as they wish about a particular topic. For example, use the first page of your Web-based report card to communicate general measures of quality (for example, overall patient satisfaction scores, nosocomial infection rates, or c-section rates). By "clicking on" a general topic area, additional pages of detailed measurement results can be viewed. Information organized in this fashion allows consumers to choose the level of detail they need to make choice decisions. The ability to sort through report card data to find what they are most interested in knowing has been consistently requested by the public.[13]

Avoid Complicated Graphics or Statistics

Visitors to the Web don't like to wait for pretty pictures—unless, of course, they're out for a Sunday afternoon joyride in cyberspace where pleasure is a priority. The best advice: Know your user and keep the graphics simple, especially on the first page of the report card where people must decide whether they wish to proceed further into the informational sections of the report. Also remember that some people have difficulty processing mathematical concepts.[14] Whatever quality measures you display should be accompanied by simply worded explanations of how these measures reflect provider performance.[15]

Develop Strong Internal Linkages and External Web Navigation

Make sure the links between pages work and that it's easy for people to get from one page of the report card to another. External links should be provided to related Web sites that are valuable to customers, and new links should be added as they become available.

Make the Report Card Fun and Interactive

Give readers an opportunity to participate in judging the quality of health care services through games, surveys, contests, and free giveaways. People want to be a part of the action. Although it's important to give customers information, they also need a chance to be involved. Visitors to the report card Web site should be given the opportunity to react to what they've learned on the site or ask questions. For example, the Kettering Medical Center in Ohio offers the public an opportunity to order written informational literature on a number of medical topics, including how to choose a doctor and a guide to choosing health plans.[16]

Offer People a Reason to Return

Develop a "what's new" box to call attention to new and upcoming features on your report card Web page. Also, consider making your site a resource for breaking national and local news about health care quality-related issues. For example, the organization may want to summarize the results from a significant new medical discovery, provide an analysis of the results, and suggest actions that consumers can take to apply the new findings to their daily lives.

For example, the Web site for the Cardiovascular Institute of the South at Duke University includes summaries of two recently published articles that suggest that hospitals where more than 200 angioplasty operations are performed annually have lower cardiac surgery mortality rates (http://www.icorp. net/cardio/articles/ang-vol.htm). Consumers are urged to find out how many angioplasty procedures are performed by their surgeon and at the hospital where they are considering having the surgery.

Deliver Value–Added, Focused Information

This is the biggest challenge in developing a Web-based provider report card. Following is a list of Web sites that have used various reporting strategies to deliver performance measurement information and advice to consumers:

- American Association of Health Plans (http://www.aahp.org)
- Arizona Department of Health Services (http://www.hs.state.az.us/)
- California Consumer Health Scope (http://www.healthscope.org)
- Community General Hospital (http://www.cgh.org/execsumm.htm)
- Connecticut Hospital Association (http://www.chime.org)
- *Detroit Free Press,* Nursing Home Ratings (http://www.freep.com/nursing/ratings.htm)
- Duke Medical Center (http://www.mc.duke.edu/patient/)
- Group Health Cooperative of Puget Sound (http://www.ghc.org)
- Healthcare Report Cards (http://www.healthcarereportcards.com)
- Healthfinder (http://www.healthfinder.gov)
- HealthPartners (http://www.healthpartners.com)
- Health Policy Resources (http://www.cmanet.org/public_interest/)
- Mayo Clinic Health Oasis (http://www.mayohealth.org)
- Stanford Medworld (http://www-med.stanford.edu/medworld)
- Utah Hospital Consumer Guide (http://hlunix.hl.state.ut.us/hda/consumer/con_97.html)

Visit these sites and determine what you like and don't like about the manner in which the organization is providing information to consumers. Don't limit yourself to health care sites only. Any well-constructed Web site can serve as a model for the provider's information-sharing strategy. For example, the Insurance News Network (http://www.insure.com) offers ratings of various health plans and other insurance companies. A report card–type grading system (A = excellent, B = good, and E = very weak) is used to communicate information to the public. Another example is the Internet Banker Scorecard produced by Gomez Advisors, Inc. (http://www.gomezadvisors. com/Banks/Scorecard/). It rates Internet banking services on five different parameters: ease of use, customer confidence, on-site resources, relationship services, and overall costs. Each banking service also receives an overall score that is an average of the scores for each of the individual parameters. A brief description of the scoring methodology accompanies the ratings.

Combine the best of what you see on the Web pages of other companies and begin to build your own Internet-based report card. Your goal should be to design an Internet-based report card that is attractive, informative, and useful and accurately portrays your professional image to consumers.

Promoting an Internet-Based Report Card

A Web site is not a "field of dreams." There is no guarantee that if you build an Internet presence, your consumers will visit your Web site. Although many health care organizations have already begun to disseminate quality-of-care information on their Web sites, consumers may not be aware these data are available. A 1996 study found that less than 1 percent of American adults indicated they'd seen quality-of-health-care information on the Internet.[17]

The main factor in successful promotion of an Internet presence is hard work and dedication to long-term results. Providers can promote their Web page using a number of methods, including the following:[18]

1. *Registering it with a popular search engine.* Registration instructions are provided at the Web site for each search engine. Statistics show that 90 to 95 percent of a Web site's search engine traffic is delivered from the top 15 search engines. (See table 3-3.) Software can help the provider automate the promotion process by offering registration in hundreds of search engines with the click of the mouse. Moreover, several promotion software packages are available on the Internet for limited-time free trials. The provider's Web site developer can use many "tricks" to help get its site noticed. META Tags, TITLE Tags, and effective usage of keywords (such as report card, quality of care, or high-quality health

Table 3-3. Popular Internet Search Engines and the Universal Resource Locators (URL)

Search Engines	Universal Resource Locators (URL)
Alta Vista	http://www.altavista.com
AOL NetFind	http://www.aol.com/netfind/
Excite	http://www.excite.com
HotBot	http://www.hotbot.com
Infoseek	http://guide.infoseek.com
LookSmart	http://www.looksmart.com
Lycos	http://www.lycos.com
Microsoft	http://home.microsoft.com
Magellan	http://www.mckinley.com
Netscape	http://www.netscape.com
Northern Lights	http://www.northernlight.com *or* http://www.nlsearch.com
Search.com	http://www.search.com
Snap	http://www.snap.com
WebCrawler	http://Webcrawler.com
Yahoo!	http://www.yahoo.com

care) throughout the site are critical to obtaining search engine exposure for its provider report card. The provider should make sure its site developer has some experience in this area.

2. *Representing the Web site as a link on another health care-related site.* A well-designed reciprocal linking strategy will cultivate traffic for the long term. This strategy can be very labor-intensive. To have reciprocal links you must contact the site you want to link from and request that it represent your site as a link on its Web site. Most organizations will be happy to accommodate you if you add their site as a link on your page.

3. *Using a traditional newspaper or magazine press release.* This can be an effective announcement for your new Internet-based report card. Don't limit press releases to the initial start-up of your Web site. Issue press releases every time a major update is made or new performance measures are added.

4. *Ensuring that the Web address is on view everywhere.* It should be evident on letterheads, faxes, business cards, invoices, and other promotional items.

The costs for Web page promotion are relatively small. Much of it can be done with a mere investment of time devoted to getting the word out. If you prefer to have a professional do it, plenty of Internet marketing companies would be happy to help. Whether you promote your report card site yourself or hire an Internet marketing company, promotion is a very important step in the process to get your report card site noticed.

Evaluating the Success of an Internet–Based Report Card Strategy

It's not enough to just create the Web site. The provider must "close the loop with an evaluation of how well the Web site is meeting its intended purpose," says Paula Swain of Swain and Associates Healthcare Consultants in St. Petersburg, Florida. Encourage visitors to your site to give feedback to the Webmaster and producers of the site. Following are several tactics to use in gathering information on how the report card site is perceived by the public and what additional information consumers would like to see on your site.

- *Formal (on-Web) inquiry.* This method consists of a form on the site that directs the reader to fill in the blanks and press the enter key or click a button to send the feedback instantly to an interested party. A form like this can be found at the Swain and Associates Web page at http://www.sna consulting.com/customers/feedback.htm.
- *Interactivity feedback.* This technique allows readers to ask questions about the content information on the site. Queries can be made to clarify or request more detail. This type of interactivity allows consumers to feel connected with the organization. Many health care organizations provide a customer service telephone number for Web visitors who would like to call for more information on the topics contained in the Web-based report card. Even when consumers have access to report card information on your Web site, some may need to consult a live person.[19] More than 40 percent of respondents to a recent Louis Harris and Associates' survey indicated it would be useful to have more opportunities for individual assistance in order to ask questions about health plan selections.[20]
- *Focus groups.* A group of community members can be called together to help evaluate the format and content of your Web-based report card. Piloting the project with a group of consumers will help ensure that you have a truly consumer-friendly report card strategy. The knowledge gained from your customers can keep you on the right track toward building a user-friendly report card.

Conclusion

A recent study of Internet usage conducted by Deloitte & Touche, Detroit, and VHA, Irving, Texas, revealed that more than one-third of Internet users regularly surf the Net for health care information.[21] Many people are seeking information on a specific disease or medical condition. With Internet popularity on the rise, the provider must consider ways of using this technology to promote quality of care, linking performance measurement data with medical information Web sites. Health care futurists agree that the Web is fast becoming a major conduit for information transfer within the health care industry and with the users of health care services.[22] Authors of a recent study that examined patients' use of public performance reports in Pennsylvania found that delivering performance information to the public may be one of the greatest challenges.[23] It was suggested that Internet-based media would be a viable dissemination strategy.

An Internet-based report card offers a provider an important opportunity to connect with consumers. With careful planning a provider can create a user-friendly report card that promotes its services while offering valuable self-help advice to consumers.

After establishing an Internet presence and beginning to share performance data with the public, the provider's message will need to be continually updated. The Web site should become a static billboard on the information superhighway. Think in terms of "the relentless pursuit of perfection." The Lexus Corporation effectively captured the notion that excellence demands a continual search for a better way. In the same way, a Web strategy should be thought of as a continual journey. The look of your Web site as well as the information contained in your report card should change in response to market conditions and feedback from your consumers.

References

1. Oregon Consumer Scorecard Consortium, *Oregon Consumer Scorecard Project,* NTIS publication no. PB97-117758 (Springfield, VA: National Technical Information Service, 1997).

2. Institute of Medicine, *Improving the Managed Care Market: Adding Choice and Protections* (Washington, DC: National Academy Press, 1996).

3. U.S. Internet Population Clock, Methodology, *Iconocast* (August 1998); WWW document, November 1998, URL: http://www.icono cast.com/methodology.html.

4. President's Advisory Commission on Consumer Protection and Quality in the Health Care Industry, *Quality First: Better Health Care for All Americans* (Washington, DC: Government Printing Office, March 1998). Copies of this report can be downloaded from the commission's World Wide Web site at www.hcqualitycommission.gov.

5. Office of Technology Assessment, *The Quality of Medical Care: Information for Consumers* (OTA-H-386) (Washington, DC: U.S. Government Printing Office, 1988).

6. College of Healthcare Information Management Executives (CHIME), Healthcare Information Technology Warehouse, Internet/ Intranet Software: An Interview with Leland Kaiser, PhD, "Question: What attitude should we have toward on-line services in healthcare?" WWW document, URL: http://warehouse.chime-net.org/software/ interintrasw/kaisar.htm.

7. President's Advisory Commission on Consumer Protection and Quality in the Health Care Industry, *Quality First: Better Health Care for All Americans* (Washington, DC: Government Printing Office, March 1998).

8. Annette Walker, "Medical Quality Report Cards: How to Get Yours on the Honor Roll. Best Practice Perspective," WWW document, April 1998, URL: http://www.best4health.com.

9. Many of these tips have been adapted from D. Goldstein and J. Florey, *Best of the Net: The Online Guide to Healthcare Management and Medicine* (New York: McGraw-Hill/Irwin Professional Publishing, 1996).

10. Oregon Consumer Scorecard Consortium, *Oregon Consumer Scorecard Project,* NTIS publication no. PB97-117758 (Springfield, VA: National Technical Information Service, 1997).

11. Mark Hochhauser, "Designing Readable Report Cards," *Managed Healthcare* 8, no. 5 (May 1996): 15–22.

12. National Center for Education Statistics, *1992 National Adult Literacy Survey* (Washington, DC: National Center for Education Statistics, 1993).

13. Research Triangle Institute, *Information Needs for Consumer Choice, Final Focus Group Report,* prepared for the Office of Research and Demonstrations, Health Care Financing Administration (Research Triangle Park, NC: RTI, 1995).

14. Office of Technology Assessment, *The Quality of Medical Care: Information for Consumers* (OTA-H-386) (Washington, DC: U.S. Government Printing Office, 1988).

15. Jeanne McGee, Shoshanna Sofaer, and B. Kreling, *Findings from Focus Groups Conducted for the National Committee for Quality Assurance Medicare and Medicaid Consumer Information Projects* (Washington, DC: National Committee for Quality Assurance, July 1996).

16. Kettering Medical Center Web site at http://www.ketthealth.com.

17. Kaiser Family Foundation and Agency for Health Care Policy and Research, "Americans as Health Care Consumers: The Role of Quality Information: Questionnaire and Toplines" (April 1997); WWW document, October 1996, URL: http://www.ahcpr.gov/research/kffhigh.htm.

18. Jamie Oikle, "IntrepidNet Marketing. So You Want to Get on the Internet: Internet Marketing" (1997), WWW document, URL: http://www.intrepidmarketing.com/Articles/getstarted.html.

19. Judith H. Hibbard and J. J. Jewett, "Will Quality Report Cards Help Consumers?" *Health Affairs* 16, no. 3 (March 1997): 218–28.

20. S. L. Isaacs, "Consumers' Information Needs: Results of a National Survey," *Health Affairs* 15, no. 4 (April 1996): 31–41.

21. 1998 Environmental Assessment, "Setting Foundations for the Millennium," Deloitte & Touche, Detroit, and VHA, Irving, TX, 1998.

22. College of Healthcare Information Management Executives (CHIME), Healthcare Information Technology Warehouse, Internet/Intranet Software: An Interview with Leland Kaiser, PhD, "Question: What attitude should we have toward on-line services in healthcare?" WWW document, URL: http://warehouse.chime-net.org\software\interintrasw/kaisar.htm.

23. Eric C. Schneider and Arnold M. Epstein, "Use of Public Performance Reports: A Survey of Patients Undergoing Cardiac Surgery," *Journal of the American Medical Association* 279, no. 20 (May 27, 1998): 1638–42.

CHAPTER FOUR

Recognizing the Legal
Issues Surrounding
Provider Report Cards

Alice G. Gosfield, Esq.

The era of public dissemination of performance data—whether based on customer satisfaction or focused on clinical outcomes—is just beginning. From a legal perspective, this means that an understanding of the legal issues surrounding public report cards published by providers cannot be based on case law because there simply is not enough experience with these initiatives to have generated lawsuits, let alone the appellate court cases that produce precedents.[1] In this newly dawning age of public, quality-focused information, assessment of these legal issues necessarily, then, turns on legal analogy and good common sense.

Public report cards for consumers can include various types of information, including the qualifications of the physicians in the hospital's network or on the medical staff, customer satisfaction with care, clinical outcomes for specific conditions, or extent of adherence to clinical practice guidelines. Although customer satisfaction is the focus of much report card reporting to date, as time goes by more clinical information will be supplied. Legal issues will arise from both types of activities, but greater peril lies in clinical data than in customer satisfaction data.

This chapter considers the types of legal issues likely to arise in this new environment and offers some commonsense tips for avoiding trouble.

Types of Legal Problems

There are two fundamental types of potential legal problems when a health care provider chooses to make public some type of quantitative information about its performance: tort liability and regulatory liability. The following sections speculate on some of the potential problems that could arise in each of these areas when health care organizations publish consumer-targeted report cards.

Tort Liability

Tort liability can arise where (1) some harm is inflicted; (2) the court finds the provider has a duty to the recipient of the information; (3) there is a breach of this duty based on a breach of the applicable standard of care; and (4) the breach caused the harm to the complainant. Following are provider report techniques that, if handled inappropriately, could result in tort liability.

Use of Customer Satisfaction Data The first potential liability will arise if a consumer, using information in a report card, claims to have been harmed as a result of reliance on that information. This issue has been raised in health plan liability suits. In *Boyd v. Einstein,*[2] the plaintiff claimed that the patient died of a pneumothorax because the gatekeeper did not refer her back to the surgeon when she reported chest pain after a breast biopsy. The court found that the HMO could be held liable because the gatekeeper was the plan's ostensible agent; but, in addition, the court specifically noted the plan's advertising in which it had said it would guarantee the quality of its care. The court noted this statement when it permitted the case to go to trial even though the plan had argued that it should not, as a matter of law, be held liable for the physician's failed decision making. Among other reasons to let the case proceed, the court considered the advertising statement an obligation of the HMO. Similarly, when a hospital publishes data that report specific outcomes for a specific procedure or treatment (for example, "95 percent of our patients are back to full functioning in two months after a knee replacement"), there is the risk that this could be seen as a contract to cure. For the patient in the 5 percent category, the reason for outlier status could be raised as an issue in a subsequent lawsuit.

Customer satisfaction data are much less troublesome if they are reported in terms of "our patients report they feel very satisfied with our care 75 percent of the time." Whether in terms of access, service, or overall satisfaction, all that is being reported is a group's perception at a specific moment in time. This very type of information is being reported on the Internet by the Minnesota integrated systems and physician groups that contract with the Buyer's Health Care Action Group.[3] Assuming the data are reported accurately, the mere fact that a specific group of patients reported more or less satisfaction is unlikely in and of itself to create legal problems. However, despite this general premise, unanticipated, novel arguments can always be crafted by clever plaintiffs counsel, depending on the nature of the harm suffered by the patient. For example, in a health plan where patients must select a specific care system or hospital (a situation that sometimes happens where integrated delivery systems take global financial risk), if a patient was misled in selecting a hospital based on customer satisfaction data and was later harmed, the inducement to enter into the relationship that led to the clinical problem could come up in litigation. Similarly, if a hospital reports that 95 percent of its medical staff members are board certified, but in fact only 80 percent are actually board certified, and 15 percent are qualified to take the board exam but are waiting for the opportunity to do so, the same issues of detrimental reliance might be raised. Nonetheless, it is clinical data that will likely form the basis for real tort problems, if any.

If a patient selects a hospital based on its published rates of mortality and he or she is harmed, one of the issues likely will be whether the hospital complied with the relevant standard of care in its publication of the data. In a case where the parties are trying to establish the standard of care, issues that may arise could include whether the hospital based its claimed success rates on only the best data or whether in reporting or advertising the results, the data were presented in a manner that misled the consumer and could have been expected to do so. Another issue might well be whether the measure of success, "We follow the National Comprehensive Cancer Network (NCCN) guidelines for treatment of breast cancer and our patients have a cure rate of 70 percent over five years," was accurately stated. Did the caregivers in fact use the NCCN guidelines and adhere to them? Was the success rate based on complete data? Were the data sufficiently current as to be meaningful?

Use of Comparative Reporting   Another type of tort liability can arise from comparative reporting—claims that refer to competitor institutions either directly or indirectly. Inaccurate statements about competitors can result in liability for business defamation. On the other hand, accurate, verifiable statements do not create such liability. Implied denigrations are somewhat less troublesome ("We have the most experienced cardiac bypass surgeons in the Metro area"), unless the statement is untrue.

Use of Superlatives in Advertising and Public Data   The use of superlatives in advertising and public data can raise a different issue. In general, the law does not require any provider to give the best care or to produce the highest quality. Rather, liability will not attach where an organization can show that it provided that level of care that a similarly situated facility acting reasonably would have provided under similar circumstances. When the hospital claims it provides the best-quality care in the community or has the best doctors on staff, it is affirmatively holding itself out as meeting a higher standard than the law would otherwise impose. Moreover, because superlatives are in their essence judgmental, comparative, and rarely based on any quantified data, they can produce liability because the determination of what is best at any given moment will depend on the status of others offering the same service.

Use of Trademarked or Copyrighted Information Yet another type of liability can arise when an organization makes use of trademarked or copyrighted information (intellectual property) by references that incorporate someone else's intellectual property or appropriate it in a way that could be misleading. These actions can lead to copyright or trademark infringement suits. For example, many hospitals and health plans are accredited. The point of accreditation is to differentiate some organizations from others. Maintenance of the integrity of the meaning of accreditation and even of the levels of accreditation is, therefore, critical to the accrediting body. Both the Joint Commission on the Accreditation of Healthcare Organizations (JCAHO) and the National Committee for Quality Assurance (NCQA)[4] publish advertising guidelines limiting the uses that may be made of references to a hospital's, network's, or health plan's accreditation. NCQA even goes so far as to dictate acceptable and unacceptable statements that may be made in advertising. Although the primary penalty for breach is loss of accreditation, for a never-surveyed, never-accredited entity to claim in a report card or advertisement that it met all standards of the accrediting body would be problematic as a matter of law.

Similarly, the NCCN publishes clinical practice guidelines on cancer treatment. Although the guidelines are published annually in the journal *Oncology,* NCCN holds the copyright on them. A hospital that claimed to use the NCCN guidelines, but, in fact, had altered them in their application in some way, would also be a potential target of legal action for copyright infringement. In addition, the NCCN name is registered and protected. So is HEDIS (the Health Plan Employer Data and Information Set), which is published by NCQA. Thus, references to NCCN or HEDIS are protected. Improper use of references to these protected marks is another form of potential liability in publishing performance data.

Regulatory Liability

Regulatory liability can rest on federal or state statutes and regulations that provide for enforcement of a hospital's obligation to behave in a certain way. In addition to private liability in the form of damages that can be assessed in a lawsuit by one person against a provider, there are also regulatory authorities relevant to hospital report card production. In some states, notably Pennsylvania and New York, public entities report data about hospitals in public report cards. Compliance with the laws on reporting to those government agencies may be an issue in those states. Of greater significance for a hospital-sponsored report card, though, are the authorities of the Federal Trade Commission (FTC) and state laws regulating advertising and unfair trade practices.

Federal Trade Commission The FTC regulates advertising in interstate commerce. Claims that are made for health products have been a focus of their interest. For example, the FTC filed an administrative complaint against Cancer Treatment Centers of America and two affiliated hospitals, which was settled by a consent agreement with no admission of wrongdoing. According to the complaint, among other issues, a version of the company's promotional brochure represented that it had statistical evidence to demonstrate that its survival rate for cancer patients was among the highest recorded. According to the complaint, the company did not have adequate evidence to back up its claims.[5] In the proposed settlement, the respondents were required to have competent and reliable evidence of a scientific nature, in certain instances, to support any representation: (1) regarding the survival or cure rates for their cancer patients or for any disease treatment they offer; (2) that any cancer treatment is approved or endorsed by any independent organization or facility; and (3) regarding the efficacy, performance, safety, or benefits of any cancer treatment. Testimonials are also problematic, but not prohibited, if they were truthful atypical testimonials that clearly and prominently disclosed in close proximity to each testimonial the generally expected results or a cautionary note that other patients should not expect similar results. The published proposed settlement is an excellent guide to the pitfalls in using data in advertising, whether or not a provider is producing data that will be used in interstate commerce (across state lines).

The FTC generally monitors the substantiation of claims made in advertising to ensure that advertisers and ad agencies have a reasonable basis for advertising claims before they are disseminated. "A firm's failure to possess and rely upon a reasonable basis for objective claims constitutes an unfair and deceptive act or practice in violation of Section 5 of the Federal Trade Commission Act."[6] The FTC also regulates comparative advertising, which is not prohibited. Even disparaging advertising is permissible as long as it is truthful and not deceptive.[7] So a hospital could publish comparative data but would have to be certain that they were accurate and truthful.

State Law   Where the FTC does not have jurisdiction because there is no interstate commerce, state laws may apply. Most states have laws regarding fair trade and business practices and unfair competition that can apply to provider report cards.

Examples of the types of behavior that violate these acts include the following:

- Representing that goods or services have sponsorship, approval, characteristics, ingredients, uses, benefits, or quantities they do not have
- Representing that goods or services are of a particular standard, quality, or grade if they are of another
- Disparaging the goods, services, or business of another by false or misleading representation of fact[8]

As with the FTC, the emphasis in these statutes is on the truth of the information presented.

How to Minimize Legal Perils

Against this background, some practical guidance is possible, even though there is not much case law to consider in determining how to proceed. For example:

- *Do not publish any report card or data without having it, and all the statements characterizing it, reviewed by legal counsel.* The potential legal implications of claims made in a report card will continue to evolve over time. Legal counsel should be involved in reviewing all such advertising or reporting to ensure that obvious problems have been anticipated and avoided.
- *Make sure there is substantiation of claims made by reviewing carefully the validity, completeness, and currency of the basis for the information to be published.* Both regulators and courts will consider carefully the substantiation and truth of claims made. Statements that could be misleading should be avoided. Testing consumer response to information before publishing it can point out potential pitfalls here. Self-selected, self-serving information that eliminates any unfavorable information from the data to be reported could be

problematic, although in advertising one always seeks to put the best light on the product.

- *Use disclaimers about the applicability of the information.* Disclaimers are intended to limit liability for applications of hospital report card data that the publisher could not anticipate. For example: "Reasonable effort has been made to ensure the accuracy of the information presented here. The hospital and its employees, agents, and staff make no representation, guarantee or warranty, express or implied, that this compilation is error free and will bear no responsibility or liability for the results or consequences of their use." Similar disclaimers include statements such as: "The information contained in this report card is not intended nor is it implied to be a substitute for professional medical advice. Always seek the advice of your physician or other qualified health provider with regard to the health services you seek and your needs."

  In the settlement noted above, the FTC sought disclaimers with respect to testimonials (much like customer satisfaction data) that would qualify the information's applicability. Something like "This information was obtained from a review of medical records of patients treated for impotence in March 1998. The cure rate presented is not a guarantee with regard to any specific individual's care" would be helpful.

- *Avoid using superlatives.* The highest rate of cure, the most qualified endocrinologists, the best physicians, the fastest return to work times should be avoided in characterizing report card data. These statements are difficult to substantiate and could be seen to be misleading. Such statements by a provider may create a contract with the patient for an outcome or, at a minimum, to hold the organization as not having provided the best care when something goes wrong later. If you want to make claims about how superlative you are, it is always better to simply reprint someone else's characterization of your activities. "Rated the best hospital for heart transplant in the metropolitan area by ABC News-paper Inc. for the last three years" would be a statement with very different legal significance from "our doctors are the best in the metropolitan area."

- *Make sure your liability insurance carrier knows what you are doing.* If you intend to get into the business of publishing performance data, it is always a good idea to let your liability carrier know you are stepping into the arena of making public claims about your performance. Because liability for defamation is often excluded from malpractice liability policies, it is important to have insurance coverage to protect you for the risks you are undertaking.

Conclusion

The era of public report cards has been launched. Although lawsuits based on these reports are not evident, legal pitfalls lurk. This article has been only a brief review of the more obvious potential legal problems that might arise. Other legal issues bear consideration in the publication of aggregate data, including the following:

- Whether confidentiality is breached when the information on which the report card is based is obtained from patients' records
- Whether it is necessary to get patient consent to access data that will be reported
- Whether an institutional review board must consider production of outcomes data to be included in a report card database
- Whether data that were collected were in fact reviewed to see if they demonstrated quality problems that should be acted on
- Whether the clinical practice guidelines that formed the measurement tool to produce the data reported were appropriately selected, developed, and applied

All of these offer potential legal perils. Whether any of these jeopardies come to pass or prove problematic is yet to be seen. Above all, however, it is important to remember that if a provider exercises due care, ensures that data are accurate, and explains their appropriate uses, liability can be diminished. In the last analysis, good insurance coverage is always helpful.

References

1. For a full consideration of legal issues pertaining to managed care quality, see Alice G. Gosfield, *Guide to Key Legal Issues in Managed Care Quality* (New York: Faulkner & Gray, 1996).

2. 547 A. 2d 1229 (Pa. Super. 1988).

3. "Money Matters: A BHCAG Update from the Twin Cities," *Business and Health* (April 1998): 41–51.

4. At the time of this writing, the author is chairman of the board of NCQA. The opinions expressed here are hers alone and should not be attributed to or imputed in any way to NCQA.

5. "Cancer Treatment Centers Settle FTC Allegations over Ad Claims," *BNA Health Law Reporter* 5 (March 21, 1996): 420.

6. FTC Policy Statement Regarding Advertising Substantiation, Appendix, *Federal Register* 48 (March 11, 1983): 10471.

7. 16 CFR 14.15(c)(1).

8. See, for example, 73 P.S. 210-2(4).

CHAPTER FIVE

Developing and Disseminating the *Michigan Hospital Report*

Mark Sonneborn, MS, CHE

The *Michigan Hospital Report,* first published in 1996, is a voluntary public service of the Michigan Health & Hospital Association (MHA). It presents performance data for virtually all Michigan short-term acute care community hospitals. The main data source for the report is the Michigan Inpatient Data Base (MIDB), which contains roughly 1.3 million individual discharge records provided to the MHA by Michigan hospitals. The two primary objectives of the report are to help Michigan hospitals improve their performance and to help consumers become better informed about health care services. Moreover, it is the goal of the MHA, as yet unrealized, to act as a catalyst in encouraging other holders of health data to share their information publicly. Within MHA and the Michigan hospital industry, the report is an affirmation of provider commitment to public accountability—one of the data principles that guide the work of the MHA.

It is the MHA's belief that there are probably many strategies for creating and distributing hospital performance measurement data to the public, and each situation has its unique set of circumstances. The report created by MHA is far from perfect—it has its detractors from both within the hospital industry and without. Any report card initiative should be viewed as a first step, with the understanding that it is expected to evolve and improve over time.

This chapter describes the experiences of MHA and its constituents in creating the *Michigan Hospital Report* (which will be referred to as the report or public report). It also discusses issues that should be addressed by all report card developers and offers advice on how to avoid potential pitfalls when creating publicly accessible health care performance reports.

Pursuing the Goal of an Integrated Health Care Database

Unlike some states, Michigan has no legislatively mandated hospital data-reporting process. In 1995, bills were introduced to the state legislature that would have established a health care database. Although the legislation appeared to call for creation of a comprehensive database, Michigan hospital leaders were concerned that the information would primarily encompass inpatient data. In a position paper issued that year, the MHA reiterated its commitment to improve the health status of Michigan's population through high-quality, efficiently delivered care and to provide information about the performance of health care providers and health plans. Although the MHA opposed adoption of legislation designed solely to collect hospital data, it supported the long-term goal of an integrated health database that would combine data from physicians, other providers, purchasers, insurers, public health departments, and other sources. It was believed that such a system would more accurately measure community health needs, allow meaningful comparisons among health plans and providers, and permit health coverage to be tailored to meet the needs of the communities being served. The MHA argued in favor of a voluntary effort, rather than a legislative mandate, to achieve this long-term goal.

The legislative effort was subsequently dropped, but the MHA continued to support creation of a comprehensive database and encouraged all holders of health care information to voluntarily report their data. As a first step toward realizing the goal of an integrated health care database, most of the Michigan acute care hospitals agreed to voluntarily report patient discharge data to the MHA to enable creation of a publicly available hospital performance report.

After the MHA board approved the concept of a public report, the first step was to identify who would be responsible for its different aspects. Initially, MHA appointed a single committee to oversee every aspect of the report. Along the way, however, it became apparent that there was a need to separate technical issues from dissemination and public relations issues. The technical work tended to be concentrated at the beginning of the process, whereas distribution issues were expected to continue throughout the project's lifetime.

A technical advisory group composed of physicians, quality management, and marketing and planning professionals from a cross-section of Michigan hospitals was assigned the task of developing the content and format of the first report. For the dissemination issues, the MHA found it helpful to form another advisory group composed of public relations specialists and MHA members.

Designing the Report

Following is a description of the key issues the technical advisory group responsible for report design and content had to confront for the initial and subsequent public reports. These same issues will need to be addressed by any group wishing to create a public report of this type. In addition to listing the key decisions that must be made, some of the lessons learned by the MHA advisory group are described below.

Selecting the Target Audience

For this public report project, consensus on the target audience was reached with relative ease. Because it was believed that large employers and insurance companies already had the resources they needed to analyze claims information, the technical advisory group thought it was most important to target the public report to consumers, a group with virtually no access to provider performance data.

It should be noted that the technical advisory committee recognized the inherent shortcomings of giving consumers information exclusively about hospitals. People are, for the most part, able to choose a health plan and a physician, whereas their choice of hospital may be limited by health plan contracts or physician preferences. Despite the fact that the public may not have direct control over their choice of hospital provider, the MHA adopted the attitude that it was necessary to start the database development process somewhere, and hospital data were perhaps the easiest to obtain.

Reviewing Examples of Other Public Reports

The technical advisory committee reviewed public reports that had been created by states such as Florida, Pennsylvania, and California, as well as regional efforts such as the Cleveland Health Quality Choice project. Much of the format and content of the initial Michigan public report were patterned after these existing models. As MHA gained experience in creating the public report and reviewed comments from its users, the Michigan report soon took on its own unique character.

Selecting Performance Measures

Length of stay (LOS) and mortality rates were chosen as the base measures for the MHA public report. These are also the most frequently reported measures in hospital report cards produced by other groups. The technical advisory group reviewed a list of the most common reasons for hospitalizations in Michigan and ultimately decided to focus the first report on cardiac care, obstetrics, and joint replacement cases. New measures, including financial information, were added with subsequent reports. Following is a list of the hospital-specific performance indicators included in the May 1998 report:

- LOS and mortality
  - —Selected medical cases
  - —Selected surgical cases
  - —Nonsurgical heart care
  - —Coronary artery bypass grafts
  - —Valve repair
- LOS only
  - —Total knee replacement
- Obstetrics
  - —Cesarean section (c-section) rate
  - —Vaginal birth after cesarean (VBAC) rate
- Financial information
  - —Case-specific Medicare payment for five most frequent reasons for admission
  - —Average Medicare reimbursement and cost of care for Medicare patients
  - —Operating margin and long-term debt-to-equity

Selecting a Severity–Adjustment Methodology

The ability to "severity adjust" patient populations was a critical element in obtaining provider acceptance of the public report. A completely separate chapter could be written on the selection of a severity-adjustment methodology. However, it is sufficient to say that a number of methodologies are available and the technical advisory group developed a set of criteria to rank the options. Reputation, technical capability, and price weighed heavily in the group's choice of the 3M All-Patient Refined Diagnosis-Related Groups (APR-DRG) system.

One of the attractive features of the APR-DRG methodology is that the system assigns a separate severity score for LOS and for risk of mortality. In other words, a patient could theoretically have a low-risk-of-mortality score and still be expected to stay in the hospital longer, thus receiving a higher severity score for LOS.

No severity system is perfect, and there are times when the APR-DRG methodology does not accurately reflect important aspects of a hospital's patient population. For example, the most common problem is that those patients with do-not-resuscitate (DNR) orders are not identified in the MIDB. Thus, the severity system treats such cases like any other and assigns a risk of mortality score that may greatly underestimate the patient's probability of death. The explanatory section of the MHA public report cautions the public that using mortality rates as an absolute gauge of the overall quality of care provided by a hospital is inappropriate because many other factors also must be considered. For example, a hospital may treat a disproportionate share of patients with DNR orders and would understandably have more deaths.

It should also be noted that the c-section and VBAC rates are not severity adjusted because, given the data set limitations of the MIDB, no suitable severity methodology for the obstetric rates could be identified.

Determining Minimum Volume Requirements

Given the MHA's data principle of public accountability, the group wanted all hospitals to have the opportunity to demonstrate their commitment to that principle. A small number of Michigan hospitals chose not to participate fully in the voluntary data-reporting program and some participating hospitals have a low volume of patients in particular categories. To reduce the effect of small numbers on performance rates, the technical advisory group established a minimum threshold of 30 annual cases for a hospital's data to be published in any one category. Also, to obtain reasonable volume numbers for smaller institutions, two groups of medical and surgical patients were consolidated for reporting purposes. The group of selected medical cases includes stroke, pneumonia, chronic lung disease, and gastrointestinal bleeding. The group of selected surgical cases includes lung surgery, lower bowel surgery, spine surgery, vascular surgery, prostate surgery, and hysterectomy.

Determining How Data Will Be Displayed

Hospitals participating in the project did not want a report that appeared to rank providers. Rather, they were more in agreement with a report format that compared each hospital's actual performance against its own expected performance. Using this methodology, the public report reveals whether an individual hospital falls within, below, or above the expected range. Differentiation among providers is only evident when, for example, hospital A is below the expected range and hospital B is within the expected range for the same performance measure. There is no statistical difference between hospitals that fall within the same range.

To produce this report, the technical advisory group used a software product called the Quality PlannerJ marketed by the Sachs Group in Evanston, Illinois. This software is able to create a unique expected range for each hospital based on its volume and severity mix as well as on statewide norms. However, the method of displaying actual performance against an expected range became somewhat controversial. The first approach that was considered was the *Consumer Reports* style, using different symbols to represent hospital performance below, above, or within the expected range. Although readers can quickly scan this type of report, MHA hospital representatives were uncomfortable with losing the depth of the information when the actual and expected range of performance were not displayed. To ensure that the public had access to the data they needed, the first public report was presented in a tabular format.

The tabular form used in the first report was found to be an overwhelming amount of numbers for readers to digest. In the second and third editions, a line graphic format was used to display the expected range and a point on the line represents the hospital's actual performance. (See figure 5-1.) Readers reacted positively to this graphic display, but it also caused the number of pages in the report to dramatically increase. Also in the third report, published in May 1998, a *Consumer Reports* style of data display was added to illustrate trends from year to year. Using a columnar format representing three years of data, each hospital's performance is illustrated with one of three different symbols that signify higher-than-expected, lower-than-expected, or as-expected performance. (See figure 5-2.)

Obtaining User Input

Ideally, the technical advisory committee should have sought feedback from the public—the target audience for the data—before proceeding with production of the first report. For a number of reasons, not the least of which were a lack of resources and a tight time schedule, MHA did not hold consumer focus group meetings before publishing the initial report. This strategy was not without risk, but it was decided that the report would be offered to the public as a first step and feedback would be solicited on how to improve future editions.

Establishing the Production Schedule

Experience has shown that there are many details to be handled from the preparation phase until the release of the report. Sometimes unexpected issues arise; for instance, an error was found in some of our software and the vendor had to repair

Figure 5-1. Excerpt from 1998 *Michigan Hospital Report*
Coronary Artery Bypass Graft Mortality, 1996
(All Michigan Hospitals)

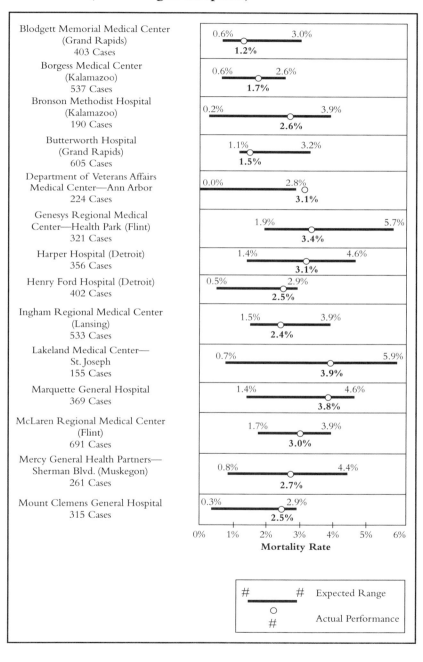

Figure 5-2. Excerpt from 1998 *Michigan Hospital Report* Three-Year Trends for LOS and Mortality Rate, 1994–96, Selected Medical Cases

Hospital Name	Length of Stay			Mortality Rate		
	94	95	96	94	95	96
Allegan General Hospital	L	L	L	○	L	○
Alpena General Hospital	○	○	●	○	○	○
Baraga County Memorial Hospital (L'Anse)	L	L	L	○	●	○
Battle Creek Health System	L	L	L	○	○	○
Bay Medical Center (Bay City)	●	●	●	○	○	○
Bell Memorial Hospital (Ishpeming)	L	L	L	○	○	○
Bi-County Community Hospital (Warren)	●	●	●	○	○	○
Bixby Medical Center (Adrian)	L	L	L	○	○	L
Blodgett Memorial Medical Center (Grand Rapids)	L	L	L	○	○	○
Bon Secours Hospital (Grosse Pointe)	●	●	●	○	○	○
Borgess Medical Center (Kalamazoo)	○	○	○	●	●	●
Borgess-Pipp Health Center (Plainwell)	L	L	L	○	○	●
Botsford General Hospital (Farmington Hills)	○	○	○	○	○	L
Bronson Methodist Hospital (Kalamazoo)	L	L	L	○	●	○
Bronson Vicksburg Hospital	L	L	L	○	○	○
Butterworth Hospital (Grand Rapids)	L	L	L	L	○	○
Carson City Hospital	L	L	○	○	○	○
Central Michigan Community Hospital (Mt. Pleasant)	L	○	L	●	○	○

● = Higher than expected	L = Lower than expected
○ = As expected	★ = Less than 30 cases

the problem before we could proceed. Plotting out tasks with their expected completion dates (building in some cushion time for unforeseen problems) is very useful for project staff. For the MHA staff, it was helpful to set a target release date first and then work backward to determine all the steps that needed to occur to meet the target date.

Producing the Report

The ease with which performance reports can be produced depends on accessibility of the data, the methods used to calculate severity-adjusted performance rates, the number of indicators included in the report, and the extent to which providers are given a prepublication opportunity to respond to the results. The steps of the report production phase for the MHA public report are listed below, along with an explanation of the process. Other groups producing provider reports may find that their production activities vary slightly.

Step 1. Draw Up a First Draft

Producing the initial MHA public report meant running the cases in the MIDB through the APR-DRG group for severity adjustment and then through the Quality PlannerJ software to establish actual and expected ranges. The MIDB contains more than 1.3 million records from more than 160 hospitals, and this sorting step took approximately one week.

Step 2. Send the Draft Report to Hospitals

Sending a prepublication version of the performance report to hospitals is viewed as a critical step in ensuring its credibility and accuracy. An element in the MHA's data release agreement is that hospitals will have at least 30 days prior to publication of any hospital-specific data to review the information. For the first report, MHA sent each of the more than

160 participating hospitals its individual results. Beginning with publication of the second report, hospitals now receive the entire report prerelease so they can view their data along with those from other hospitals.

Hospitals are asked to review and verify their data. This is somewhat problematic because most of the hospitals do not have a patient severity–adjustment system or, if they do, it may not be the APR–DRG system. However, hospitals are able to verify their actual results. They also are offered the opportunity to comment on any results that might be perceived as unacceptable by the public (for example, actual performance appeared unfavorable when compared to expected performance). If they choose, hospitals can submit a remark to explain individual variances in a specific measurement category. By imposing a 50-word limit to these comments, MHA has been able to publish the hospital's remarks at the bottom of the page on which the data appear in the report. Some hospitals use this opportunity to publicize their successes. For example, in the May 1998 public report, LOS for patients undergoing hip replacement at Mount Clemens General Hospital was shown to be well within the expected range. However, the hospital chose to add the following comment: "The length of stay at Mount Clemens General Hospital has decreased 2.4 days since 1994 due to: (1) patients' central location; (2) case management program; (3) prehospitalization education; and (4) aggressive pre/post hospitalization home care services."[1]

After hospital comments and corrections are received by the MHA, the report is updated to reflect necessary changes or additions. At this point, the work of typesetting and report design has already begun. Finalizing the report is a matter of adding a few explanatory remarks or data corrections.

Step 3. Print the Report

Sending the report to the printer is a relatively mundane task, but because it takes a couple of weeks to turn around the order, this step should be figured into the production schedule. The number of copies to be printed is an issue that should have already been decided in the dissemination discussions (see below). Likewise, printing and postage costs (if a mailing is planned) need to be factored into the report card budget. If the report will also be posted to an Internet site, staff can begin serious preparation of the on-line material at this step in the production process.

Disseminating the Report

Discussions surrounding report dissemination should begin as soon as possible after the commitment has been made to produce a publicly available performance report. If critical decisions can be made during the strategic planning phase, report production delays can be minimized. Public relations specialists should be included in the discussions. These professionals can help design a customer-friendly dissemination strategy that meets the goals of the project. The following sections address the distribution questions that need to be answered and discuss the way the MHA dissemination advisory group approached each issue.

What Does 'Public' Mean to the Provider?

This is a decision that can be made fairly early in the process and should be based on the target audience for the report. The MHA's target audience was the general public, and it was determined this audience would first hear about the report through the media. Therefore, the MHA dissemination strategy was largely aimed at the media.

To be certain the *Michigan Hospital Report* meets everyone's criteria for "publicly available," copies are sent to all depository libraries in Michigan, a selected group of print and electronic media contacts, all legislators, key trade association and business coalition executives, and any consumer who requests a copy. The initial printed report was made available to the public free of charge. However, with the second edition, people ordering the printed version were charged $10, which increased to $25 with the third edition. This charge, along with an expected declining interest in the report, allows MHA to print fewer copies. Complimentary copies continue to be sent to libraries, the media, and legislators.

It was also decided that the report would be put on the MHA's Internet Web site to increase public access to the report. Suffice it to say that the Internet version of the public report gets a lot of hits. MHA has found the Internet to be an effective dissemination tool for the report, having received many positive comments about it and even a praiseful letter to the editor in one of the state's local daily newspapers. The complete report continues to be available on the MHA's Internet site (http://www.mha.org).

What Should Be Included in Media Presentations?

One of the success factors for the public report has been the unified message that MHA and Michigan hospitals have communicated about what the report is and what it says. Working with public relations specialists, MHA and its members developed key messages to accompany the public report with supporting talking points for hospitals. Suggested responses to tough reporter questions are also developed. Of course, each hospital has to understand the reasons behind its own performance results to respond to media and public questions effectively.

The MHA prepares hospitals for potential media coverage by sending them a packet of materials that includes key messages, press releases, sample letters to the editors, and sample questions and answers. Meetings are held with constituents to provide more in-depth training for those who will be personally responsible for responding to the media.

How Should the Report Be Released to the Public?

How the report is released goes a long way toward determining how much media attention is received. Because the media are viewed by the MHA as the primary connection to the report's target audience, news coverage is vital. For the first report, the media were notified of the press conference roughly one week in advance of publication. People who attended the press conference were promised they would receive a copy of the report the day before it was released and the rest of the media would get their copy in the mail the next day. This strategy worked to our benefit, as we hosted a large number of reporters at the initial press conference.

With the second edition, a small number of reporters were invited to conduct individual interviews with MHA staff and local hospital representatives. The remaining media received a mailed press release and a copy of the report. For the third edition, a press conference was again held. The community benefits survey results, hospital financial reports, and trend data that were added to the third edition generated a lot of renewed media interest in the hospital performance report.

Measuring Success

The primary objectives of the performance report are to help Michigan hospitals improve their performance and to help consumers become better informed about health care services. To evaluate whether these objectives are being realized, the MHA conducts several evaluation activities.

The trend data included in the third edition of the *Michigan Hospital Report* provide a first-time look at how individual hospital and statewide performance rates may have changed since publication of the first report in May 1996. However, these data do not yet reflect performance changes that can be attributed to publicly available performance reports. Due to the data collection lag, the initial 1996 edition included data from 1994. The third edition published in May 1998 included 1996 performance data. It will be a few more years before the impact of public reports on hospital performance can be accurately and objectively measured.

Whether the reports add significantly to the public's knowledge about hospitals is an element that has received considerable attention by the MHA. Several activities, listed below, have been under way since the first report was published in 1996 to determine its impact on the public.

• *Assess media reaction.* Experience has shown that the report creates a one-day headline; few follow-up stories are written. Remembering that the target audience's first contact with the report is through the media, it is important to review the articles that are written to see how the message was interpreted by reporters. Nearly all the stories written about the MHA public reports have been positive and accurate.

• *Survey hospitals.* Following release of each edition, hospitals are surveyed to determine how people responded to the data. It is important to find out how the report was received by key audiences, such as the board of trustees, the medical staff, employees, and the community. Through this survey process, potentially correctable problems can be identified.

The survey process is also used to find out if the report is leading to improvements in care, given that this is a primary reason for participating in the initiative. MHA has been made aware of several anecdotal improvements in which the report was a catalyst for change. These improvements range from hospital initiatives to correct medical record documentation and coding inadequacies to communication breakthroughs between hospital administration and the medical staff. The sharing of success stories reinforces the value of the report for all hospitals.

- *Survey readers.* A formal survey is used to obtain feedback from the target audience. Following release of the first report in 1996, MHA mailed a survey to people who had ordered a hard copy of the report. The 50 percent response rate helped to provide some valuable information. One noteworthy item was that the average age of the person responding to the survey was 60. From this information, MHA surmised that a large portion of the people requesting a copy of the report did so because they were likely to be requiring some type of health care services in the near future. A feedback survey form was inserted into the 1997 and 1998 reports (figure 5-3) and is also available on the MHA Internet Web site. Report users are encouraged to complete the survey and forward it to the MHA.

The MHA has made changes to the process of report preparation and the report itself after receiving input from both readers and hospitals. The preparation phase for the next report starts immediately after the release. One might assume that the second time is smoother and more streamlined than the first, and this is true to some extent. However, because improvements are made to the report based on postrelease feedback, some elements of the process and the report itself are constantly undergoing revision. For example, the MHA has refined and redefined the performance measures each year and has developed additional tools for hospitals to use in evaluating their data during the prerelease review step.

Another phenomenon that may occur with each subsequent release of the report is a decline in the public's interest, making it less newsworthy to the media. After a few more years, the MHA will evaluate whether consumers and providers still find the information useful. If not, the MHA board will reevaluate the original premise for the report to determine how best to continue helping patients, families, and purchasers of health care be informed consumers.

Figure 5-3. 1998 *Michigan Hospital Report* Feedback Survey

Thank you for your interest in the third *Michigan Hospital Report*. Please take a couple of minutes to complete this brief survey, which seeks your opinions and suggestions about the report, and will help improve future editions. Your responses are strictly confidential. Please return this to the address on the back of the survey.

1. How did you become aware of the report?
   a. ____ Newspaper
   b. ____ Radio
   c. ____ TV
   d. ____ From your local hospital
   e. ____ Local library
   f. ____ Internet
   g. ____ Other. Please explain:_____

2. Why did you want to see this report?
   a. ____ I or a loved one needs health care.
   b. ____ As an employer, I want information to help make informed health care purchasing decisions.
   c. ____ I am a researcher.
   d. ____ I work for a health care provider.
   e. ____ I am interested in how my local hospital fared in the report.
   f. ____ Other. Please explain:_____

3. Did you read the section on Hospital Performance Data?
   ____ yes   ____ no (if no, go to 4)

   The information was:
   __ very useful __ somewhat useful __ not very useful __ not useful
                                                              at all

   Interpreting the graphs in the Hospital Performance Data section was:
   __ very easy __ somewhat easy __ somewhat difficult __ very
                                                           difficult

   Comments on the Hospital Performance Data:
   _____
   _____

4. Did you read the section on Community Benefits?
   ____ yes ____ no (if no, go to 5)

   How useful was the information in the Community Benefits section?
   __ very useful __ somewhat useful __ not very useful __ not useful
                                                              at all

Figure 5–3. (Continued)

> **Comments on the Community Benefits section:**
> _____
> _____
>
> 5. **Did you read the section on Selected Financial Indicators?**
>   ___ yes ___ no (if no, go to 6)
>
>   **How useful was the information in the Financial section?**
>   __ very useful __ somewhat useful __ not very useful __ not useful
>   at all
>
>   **Interpreting the tables in the Financial section was:**
>   __ very easy __ somewhat easy __ somewhat difficult __ very
>   difficult
>
>   **Comments on the Financial section:**
>   _____
>   _____
>
> 6. **Overall, how useful did you find the report?**
>   __ very useful __ somewhat useful __ not very useful __ not useful
>   at all
>
> 7. **If you were designing this report, what other information would be in it?**
>   _____
>   _____
>
> 8. **Please complete the following demographic questions:**
>   _____ Year of birth
>   _____ Male
>   _____ Female
>   _____ County you live in
>   _____ Zip code
>
> 9. **Comments:**
>   _____
>   _____
>   _____
>
> Please return this survey to:
>
>   Attention: Mark Sonneborn
>   Michigan Health & Hospital Association
>   6215 W. St. Joseph Highway
>   Lansing, Michigan 48917
>
> Or you may fax it to: 517-323-0946

Conclusion

Designing and disseminating provider performance measurement data require careful planning, attention to the concerns of the providers whose performance is being reported and to the target audience, and a mechanism to ensure ongoing improvement based on user feedback. The choices made by the MHA in preparing and disseminating the last three annual *Michigan Hospital Reports* have resulted in a reasonably well-accepted hospital performance measurement tool. It is hoped that by sharing these experiences, other groups will be better prepared to meet the increasing data demands of the public.

What continues to be an information void in Michigan as well as other states is the lack of performance reports for other health care entities. One of the initial goals of the MHA public report initiative was to encourage other sectors of health care to follow the lead of Michigan hospitals. Data contributed by physicians, insurance companies, employers, home health agencies, nursing homes, and other groups could help present a comprehensive and consumer-helpful picture of health care in Michigan. On a percentage basis, hospital inpatient care represents only about 25 percent of the health care dollars spent in Michigan. Hospital performance data address only a fraction of the health care delivery system. Michigan's hospitals and health systems believe in public accountability in high-quality health care. Unless other groups begin to produce their own public data reports, consumers will continue to have a very narrow understanding of the performance issues affecting their health care delivery choices.

Reference

1. Michigan Health & Hospital Association, *Michigan Hospital Report* (Lansing, MI: MHA, May 1998), p. 138.

PART TWO

Measuring Provider Performance

CHAPTER SIX

Gathering Satisfaction Data to Share with the Public

J. Mac Crawford, RN, MS, PhD
John F. Sena, PhD

Health care consumers have clearly indicated that patient satisfaction data are an important source of information about the quality of health care services.[1] Recognizing this fact, many of the health plan report cards published in the early 1990s included satisfaction measures.[2] By 1995, it was estimated that more than 95 percent of health maintenance organizations (HMOs) and 55 percent of preferred provider organizations (PPOs) were using consumer surveys to monitor care.[3] Many of these groups used satisfaction data in marketing activities. Measures of consumer satisfaction have been incorporated into the Medicare and Medicaid performance evaluation requirements, prompting the development of a standardized assessment tool. The Consumer Assessments of Health Plans Study (CAHPS), funded by the Agency for Health Care Policy and Research, has produced an integrated set of carefully tested and standardized survey questionnaires that can be used by health plans to collect information from health plan enrollees about their experiences.[4] The CAHPS survey process has been incorporated into the Health Plan Employer Data and Information Set (HEDIS), a core set of health plan performance measures developed by the National Committee for Quality Assurance.[5]

Following in the footsteps of health plans, some health care providers have begun to report satisfaction data to the public. In 1996, Mercy Hospital Medical Center in Des Moines, Iowa, distributed its first "Mercy Quality Care Report." This report, available on the Mercy Hospital Web site (http://www.mercy desmoines.org), uses bar graphs to display performance data on average charges, patient volume, length of stay, results of new treatment procedures, and patient satisfaction data. Patient satisfaction survey results from Cedars Sinai Comprehensive Cancer Center (CSCC) can be found in the November 1996 issue of its *Cancer News* newsletter, which is posted on the CSCC Web site at http://www.cscc.newslett/patsur95.htm. The center's report of satisfaction ratings uses a combination of graphic displays, narrative descriptions, and anonymous patient comments to communicate information to the public. Many health care providers throughout the country have developed, or are in the process of developing, similar report cards for distribution to the public via the Internet and print media.

Traditionally, providers have used customer satisfaction data solely for internal improvement purposes. Now that satisfaction data are being made available to the public, providers must work harder to ensure that the information they are collecting and reporting is meaningful and reliable. Methods for measuring patient satisfaction have been developing over the span of many years. Abdellah and Levine[6] weighed in with their development of scales to measure patient satisfaction with nursing care, and Rice and others[7] contributed an instrument to evaluate patient care in nursing wards. Houston and Pasanen[8] reported on patient perceptions of hospital care, and Ware[9] addressed methodological issues, such as the tendency of some respondents to answer positively regardless of their true opinion. The technological revolution made possible the handling of very large databases, and, concomitantly, entities focused on measuring patient satisfaction came into existence, grew, and multiplied in the 1980s and 1990s.

Health care is a complex industry, with services provided in treatment settings ranging from home health to intensive care. This complexity and variation in settings require careful planning of any effort to measure patient satisfaction. This chapter explains how to conduct surveys that gather worthwhile data on patient satisfaction with health care encounters. It provides guidelines for planning and implementing patient satisfaction studies and for analyzing and interpreting health care consumer-based data.

How to Conduct a Health Care Satisfaction Survey

Following are six basic steps to conducting a survey of patients' service satisfaction.

1. Establish goals and select a survey approach based on these goals.
2. Determine the broad concepts to be measured and develop survey questions.
3. Construct the survey instrument.
4. Test survey validity.
5. Administer the survey.
6. Analyze survey results.

Step 1. Establish Goals and Select an Approach

Before embarking on a satisfaction study, there should be very clear expectations of what data will be collected and how they will be used to improve care.[10] One must also consider what treatment settings are of interest. Patients who received services in the hospital, outpatient area, emergency room, physician office, or home setting are likely to have different perceptions and concerns related to their satisfaction with the visit. Survey instruments and techniques must be tailored to fit the particular setting.

Other issues to consider are options to profile individual caregivers and service sites, how many patients to interview (for example, census sampling in which all discharges are surveyed versus a smaller sample), and how many resources the organization is prepared to devote to the project. The simplest survey would consist of a preestablished number of questionnaires being mailed to a sample of discharges once per year. A more complex design would call for samples of discharges to be drawn and interviewed once per quarter.

Step 2. Determine Broad Concepts and Develop Questions

The satisfaction survey will include questions that are expected to provide information about patients' opinions, feelings, or knowledge concerning broad concepts or "constructs." For example, when surveying patients about their satisfaction with a recent hospital stay, one construct might be nursing care, another might be physician care, and yet another might be environmental factors such as room cleanliness or food service. Individual questions used for measurement of constructs can be combined to form subscales or overall scales. Which broad concepts are included in the survey should be based on the provider's goals and the questions it wants answered. Following are the most common constructs included in consumer satisfaction surveys of health care providers:

- Overall quality and satisfaction
- Interpersonal aspects of care
- Communication or information giving
- Timeliness of services
- Intention to recommend provider to others

- Technical aspects of care
- Time spent with caregivers
- Access and availability of services
- Intention to use provider again
- Satisfaction with outcomes of care
- Physical environment

Figure 6-1 provides an example of a survey instrument for measuring satisfaction with an inpatient hospital stay. The survey is divided into the following seven distinct conceptual units (constructs):

1. Issues of convenience or time
2. Environmental issues such as cleanliness
3. One or more questions about food
4. Nursing care
5. Physician care
6. Information received about medications and home care
7. Overall measures of satisfaction (including intention to recommend the hospital to family and friends)

The remaining questions may be used in analyzing the results to remove or reduce variability in overall satisfaction that may be attributed to patient differences (for example, older patients are generally more satisfied than younger ones, so this can confound the analysis). The survey also includes space for verbatim comments. Narrative comments can be a good source of ideas for improvement opportunities. Like the Cedars Sinai Cancer Center, providers may wish to excerpt positive comments to include in publicly available performance reports.

Step 3. Construct the Survey Instrument

A well-designed survey tool can produce an invaluable amount of information. Conversely, survey instruments that

Figure 6-1. Sample Questionnaire for Measuring Patient Satisfaction with Hospital Stay

This survey is about your satisfaction with your recent inpatient stay at
_____ Hospital. All responses are confidential and
anonymous. Thinking of your <u>most recent</u> stay in the hospital, please
answer the following questions.

	Strongly Disagree	Disagree	Neutral	Agree	Strongly Agree	Not Applicable
1. Finding the hospital was easy.	—	—	—	—	—	—
2. The length of time we had to wait, from the time we got to the hospital until the time I was admitted, was acceptable.	—	—	—	—	—	—
3. The waiting area was clean.	—	—	—	—	—	—
4. My room was clean.	—	—	—	—	—	—
5. The food tasted good.	—	—	—	—	—	—
6. The nurses treated me with respect.	—	—	—	—	—	—
7. The nurses answered my questions in a way I understood.	—	—	—	—	—	—
8. The nurses responded to my requests quickly.	—	—	—	—	—	—
9. The nurses spent enough time with me.	—	—	—	—	—	—
10. Overall, I was satisfied with the quality of care I received from the nurses.	—	—	—	—	—	—

Figure 6-1. (Continued)

11. The doctors treated me with respect.   — — — — — —

12. The doctors explained my treatment in a way I understood.   — — — — — —

13. The doctor spent enough time with me.   — — — — — —

14. I had confidence in the doctors' technical skills.   — — — — — —

15. Overall, I was satisfied with the quality of care I received from the doctors.   — — — — — —

16. I understood how I was supposed to care for myself at home.   — — — — — —

17. I received enough information about the medicine prescribed for me.   — — — — — —

18. I would recommend _____ Hospital to family and friends.   — — — — — —

19. Overall, I was satisfied with my most recent stay at _____ Hospital.   — — — — — —

20. Before my most recent inpatient stay, I would have described my health as being:

    Poor   Fair   Good   Very Good   Excellent

21. Currently, I would describe my health as being:

    Poor   Fair   Good   Very Good   Excellent

22. What were the month and year of your most recent visit? (Example: 01/98)
    _____ / _____

23. What is your age? _____   24. What is your gender? _____

25. Do you have any comments? _____

_____

are poorly constructed may result in low response rates or misleading information. An aesthetically pleasing layout, uncramped print, and plenty of space for appropriate answers are crucial in maintaining respondents' compliance and interest.[11] (The fine details of questionnaire design are beyond the scope of this chapter. For a readable discussion of this topic, see *Improving Survey Questions* by F. Fowler.[12]) The provider might consider using the professional services of a survey development company if its in-house people do not have experience in questionnaire layout.

Step 4. Test Survey Validity

After the provider has the tool to measure patient satisfaction, it needs to consider how well this tool measures the attitudes it is supposed to. This consideration falls under the general heading of validity and is an important component in planning and implementing any survey.

Three common forms of validity must be considered in the development of a patient satisfaction survey: content validity, construct validity, and external validity.

- *Content validity.* This is a subjective measure of how appropriate questionnaire items seem (for example, do the items make sense to the reader?). Content validity is inspected both on an overall basis (does the questionnaire as a whole make sense?) and on a subscale-specific basis (do the questions included in the different subscales seem to measure the broad concept of the construct?). The content validity of satisfaction surveys may be assessed through focus groups with former patients, as well as with the organization's staff, to ensure that all information about important concepts/ content areas are captured.[13]
- *Construct validity.* This is a measure of how components within a scale group together and relate to other components within the scale. Items that make up individual sub-

scales should correlate highly with each other. However, different subscales should not correlate highly with each other because different subscales are supposedly measuring separate underlying constructs that are assumed to act independently of each other. For example, responses to physician satisfaction and nurse satisfaction questions, two of the constructs identified in the questionnaire in figure 6-1, are presumed to be independent of each other. If these constructs were not felt to be independent, there would be little justification for creating separate subscales for both physician and nurse satisfaction. Instead, a common scale could have been used.

Researchers frequently use factor analysis and correlation analysis in assessing construct validity. Factor analysis is initially run to group variables into subscales that have maximum explanatory power. This subscale structure is checked for content validity as described above and to assess the degree to which subscales identified match those identified in previous research. Next, the internal reliability of the subscales is assessed by using Cronbach's alpha, a measure of how well different items group together in explaining a single construct.[14] Alpha values greater than .70 are commonly considered acceptable. Finally, the relationship between different subscales is investigated using correlation analysis to make sure that the factor analysis did an appropriate job of separating out underlying constructs. Here researchers expect to see that subscales do not correlate highly with each other and are therefore considered independent.

- *External validity.* This refers to the degree to which the subjects sampled for a study represent the larger population from which they came.[15] External validity can be affected by the sampling scheme used and the survey response rate. For example, if there is a very low response rate, it is quite possible that those who did not respond differed in meaningful ways from those who did. To the extent that the survey did not capture the opinions of those not responding, the survey results cannot be generalized to the entire target population.

Consulting with an expert in validity-testing techniques (known as psychometrics) is strongly recommended for new patient satisfaction surveys or when the organization is administering an established survey to a group of people who are very different from those the survey was originally designed for.

Step 5. Administer the Survey

Patient satisfaction surveys can be self-administered (mailed or completed while services are being received) or interviewer-administered (telephone or face-to-face). The choice of survey administration methods is often influenced by cost, level of desired accuracy, types of questions to be asked, and ease of conducting the survey.

- *Self-administered surveys.* These tend to be among the most common methods used by providers to gather satisfaction data. Self-administered surveys generally need to be shorter in length to encourage response. Surveys that are completed at the point-of-service and returned at the end of the encounter are among the least expensive to administer. Mailed surveys are also relatively low cost; however, the expense can increase if telephone follow-up or repeat mailings are conducted. The primary drawback of mailed surveys is the low response rates, especially when no follow-up reminders (mail or telephone) are provided.
- *Interviewer-administered surveys.* To obtain a higher survey response rate and gather a large amount of data in a short time frame, consider conducting interviewer-administered surveys. These can be done as telephone surveys or in face-to-face interviews. Both techniques require interviewer training and staff time, which can increase costs. However, interviewer-administered surveys can be somewhat longer

and more detailed than mail questionnaires, making it possible to obtain larger amounts of information.

The goals established at the start of the project, the target population, and the questions to be asked will influence survey administration decisions. In addition, the provider's available resources must also be taken into consideration. Researchers at the Health Outcomes Institute in Bloomington, Minnesota, have developed cost estimates for administering various health outcomes measurement surveys.[16] According to these researchers, the per-respondent cost for self-administered on-site surveys is $5 to $10, while mail survey administration costs range from $10 to $20. Interviewer-administered surveys are considerably more expensive, with telephone surveys costing $20 to $40 and face-to-face interviews costing $40 to $80 per respondent. The costs of administering a more simplistic patient satisfaction survey are likely to be less than the dollar estimates for gathering health outcomes study data. However, you can generally expect the per-respondent cost to go up if you want to achieve high response rates or obtain extremely detailed patient satisfaction responses.

Step 6. Analyze Survey Results

Analysis of the satisfaction survey results requires that the data be coded, entered into a database, verified, and then analyzed.

1. *Coding the data.* Data coding involves assigning a value to each response in a question. For example, the survey in figure 6-1 allows five different level-of-agreement responses to each statement, plus a response of "not applicable." The first response choice, strongly disagree, can be coded "1," the second response choice, disagree, can be coded "2," and so on. Failures to provide any answer at all for a question are inevitable and a standard code for "missing" data (such as "99") should be given to any question for which no

answer was provided. A different code (such as "55") should be used for "not applicable" responses to distinguish this response from missing responses. Alpha characters can also be used as a coding scheme to represent responses. For example, "strongly disagree" can be coded as "SD," "disagree" as "D," and so on. An alpha code such as "MR" could be used for missing responses.

2. *Entering the data.* Any number of computer database programs can be used to facilitate this step. It is quite likely that health care facilities with fairly sophisticated information systems will have already purchased database software packages such as Foxpro or Access. Smaller entities with proportionally limited budgets may want to use a product offered by the Centers for Disease Control and Prevention (CDC) in Atlanta known as Epi Info. This software package is available free of charge (there is a charge of $30 if a soft-bound manual is desired) and allows the user to easily create a data-entry template. The package also allows for simple, and some fairly sophisticated, analyses. The software may be downloaded from the Internet by setting a Web browser to http://www.cdc.gov/publications.htm. In some instances, depending on facility budgets and the scope of the project, hiring an outside vendor to do the data entry and statistical analyses may be the most appropriate course of action.

3. *Verifying the data.* Proper preparation of data for analysis is critical in ensuring accurate and meaningful results. Remember the adage, "garbage in/garbage out." If there are no data-entry checks, invalid codes can be entered into the database. The researcher must be knowledgeable about the information that should be contained in the database so that invalid codes can be identified and eliminated (for example, a value of seven on a scale that only goes from one to five). It may be necessary to clean the data by programming the computer to count all invalid data-entry codes as missing. In addition to looking for invalid codes,

data preparation should be done to find and correct logical inconsistencies in the data (for example, in one question a patient indicates that he had no contact with a nurse practitioner and in another question he rates satisfaction with the nurse practitioner as being high). Data-entry inaccuracies are harder to identify. It may be necessary to double-enter the survey results to increase the accuracy of the information in the database. Figure 6-2 lists considerations in preparing data for analysis.[17]

4. *Analyzing the data.* Analysis should begin with the careful examination of means and standard deviations of continuous variables, such as age, and frequencies and percentages of categorical variables, such as race. Usually, satisfaction items, measured on a one-to-five scale for example, can be considered continuous, interval data. That is, the difference between a one and a two is the same as the difference between a four and a five. The simplest form of analysis is to determine whether there are any important patterns in

Figure 6-2. Important Steps to Take in Preparing a Data Set for Analysis

- Study the questionnaire carefully and become familiar with questions and response scales.
- Develop a codebook linking variable names with questions.
- Verify that the number of observations ("cases") matches the number of completed questionnaires returned.
- Make decisions about which cases to retain for analysis (e.g., only cases from a certain time period may be of interest, so analysis should be restricted to those observations).
- Look for out-of-range values by running means and standard deviations (this will reveal miscoded or suspiciously unusual data values such as an age of 150).
- Look for missing data and the necessity for recodes by running frequencies and percentages (i.e., make sure variables are coded correctly and that variables with missing data will not be included in analyses).
- Keep notes of steps taken in the analysis process and save computer printouts to document the process.

Source: Larry Sachs, senior statistician, Research Department, Healthcare Research Systems, Columbus, OH, 1998.

the results and look at relationships between variables. Descriptive statistics can be used to answer such questions as "How many people strongly agreed with the statement, 'I understood how I was supposed to care for myself at home'?" At this stage it might also be instructive to examine the correlations in the data. This refers to the degree to which variables are related to each other. For example, "Who thought the hospital was easier to find, people over the age of 65 or those 65 years of age and younger?"

It may be necessary to use statistical tests to determine if the results are different from what might be expected by chance alone. For example, if the average level of overall satisfaction for a three-month period was 3.5 on a five-point scale and that average went up to 3.9 the following quarter, it would be reasonable to ask if this was a "real" increase or if it was due entirely to the fact that another sample of discharged patients was selected. More details about statistical hypothesis testing is beyond the scope of this chapter, but suffice it to say that there are many possible ways to assess significance of differences, depending on the particular variables under study.

Advanced statistical techniques such as factor analysis and multiple linear regression may be used to establish which dimensions of care are most important in overall satisfaction. Factor analysis uses the correlational relationships among variables and determines, along with the professional judgment of the researcher, which variables should "go together" to create an overall satisfaction index of some construct. Recall that one construct might be nursing care, which could be assessed with several questions. Taking an average of all of these questions produces what is known as an "overall indicator score." This score can then be used with other such scores (for example, physician care, the admission process, the discharge process, and so on) in regression equations to establish which dimensions of care appear to influence patients' overall satisfaction with care.

Collection and analysis of satisfaction survey results are only a piece of the performance improvement process. The critical next step is to summarize the results for internal and external audiences. Within the organization, patient satisfaction survey results are used to target areas for improvement. The issues of how much information is shared with the public and in what fashion are addressed by other chapters in this book.

Qualitative Measures of Patient Satisfaction

Thus far, this chapter has focused on quantitative methods of patient satisfaction measurement. For a number of reasons it is sometimes preferable to gather qualitative data. Qualitative data are obtained by soliciting in-depth information from much smaller consumer populations known as focus groups.

Advantages of Focus Groups

Focus groups have become an increasingly popular means of collecting data about consumer opinions and attitudes. The popularity of this data-gathering technique may be due to a variety of factors, including the following:

- As the pace of change increases, health care organizations need information more quickly than at any time in the past. Focus groups can be assembled and conducted, with a report on an administrator's desk, within two or three weeks.
- With financial belt-tightening an almost universal phenomenon, focus groups are generally less expensive than conducting quantitative research.
- Global patient satisfaction data are becoming less useful than data on individual services or activities. Focus groups lend themselves to exploring in detail and in depth specific behaviors, activities, issues, and problems.
- Quantitative questions are generally close-ended; the interviewee can only respond within fixed limits. Focus groups, on

the other hand, allow caregivers to explore the "why" behind the "what" of descriptive quantitative scores; to examine in-depth issues suggested by numerical scores; to probe deeply into the reactions, thoughts, and opinions of patients; to delve beneath the veneer; and to benefit from the collective wisdom of the group in determining solutions to problems.

• Focus groups contain a social dimension not present in quantitative surveying. Participants enjoy interacting with one another, exchanging ideas, and hearing about the experiences of others. Often a synergy takes place that is impossible to achieve with quantitative surveying. Many of the most sophisticated and useful ideas arise when participants piggyback on each other's comments, share ideas, challenge one another, and draw each other out. The results of the discussion are often, then, greater than the sum of its parts.

When to Use Focus Groups

The range of health care topics that can be examined and discussed by focus groups is virtually limitless. Focus group participants can be asked to describe what they think a hospital lobby should look like, advise where a physician practice should be located, evaluate strengths and weaknesses of specific hospital programs, discuss billing problems, and probe race relations issues. Although the potential topics to be explored are limited only by the organization's needs and imagination, focus groups are particularly useful in the following situations:

• Consumer opinions are needed as a starting point to plan a larger undertaking. When constructing a patient satisfaction survey, for instance, market research firms will generally conduct a series of focus groups to determine what issues or dimensions of health care are most important to patients and thus should be explored.

• In-depth information is needed to explain or clarify quantitative patient satisfaction data.

- Data are needed to corroborate or deny quantitative patient satisfaction survey findings.
- In-depth and diverse information is needed to explain complex issues or attitudes—why, for instance, a health care provider has a negative image within the community it serves.
- The thoughts and opinions of a particular, homogeneous group are desired. A hospital, for instance, may wish to know if interpersonal communication is a problem with non-English-speaking patients or if women are satisfied with the obstetrics department.
- The format and content of publicly available provider report cards require evaluation.

Focus groups work optimally when their research goals are well defined, concrete, and specific. They tend to work less well when discussing broad or amorphous topics, such as the general quality of care at a hospital or global staff problems. Focus groups can be used to identify and solve problems by providing information that may be transformed into action plans. They are, at their best, both diagnostic and therapeutic.

Focus Group Myth and Reality

With the popularity of focus groups on the rise, health care providers have developed preconceived notions about how such groups are formed and conducted. Following are some of the common myths or misconceptions about focus groups and the facts or reality surrounding them:

- *Focus groups should consist of randomly selected patients.* The reality is that the composition of the group depends on the research goals. If a health care organization desires, for instance, to probe an issue from the perspective of a specific racial, ethnic, or religious group, obviously members of that particular group should be targeted for participation. If an organization wishes to explore problem areas, it would be advisable to select patients or families of patients who expressed criticism of their health care.

- *Twelve to 15 people is an ideal size for a focus group.* The reality is that many successful focus groups have consisted of 12 to 15 members—enough people to glean valuable information, yet not too many to stifle conversation. There is nothing sacrosanct, however, about this size. In recent years the trend has been to assemble smaller focus groups, which allows for more in-depth conversation and analysis.

- *Successful focus groups depend to a large extent on the quality of the recording and filming equipment, devices such as one-way mirrors, and technical support personnel.* The reality is that the moderator, not elaborate equipment, is the key to success. Focus group accomplishments should be measured by the quality of the discussion, the depth of the probing, and the ability of the moderator to stay on-task while helping people feel free to express their opinions.

- *Lively focus groups yield better data than boring groups.* The reality is that although most people would rather be a member or observer of an energetic, vibrant group, there is no correlation between the liveliness of the group and the richness and usefulness of the data yielded. Quietness and reticence are not indications of a lack of intelligence or insight, and a restrained, calm group is not a sign of a failed endeavor.

- *Men and women should not be in the same focus group.* The reality is that unless the topic under discussion is gender-specific (such as obstetric or gynecological issues), there is no reason why men and women should not be asked to participate in the same focus group. It is the responsibility of the moderator to draw remarks from each group and not allow one gender to dominate. One of the benefits of having a gender mix is that it will become evident if men and women see an issue differently. Women, for instance, may be more interested in the convenience and lighting of the parking area, while men may be more concerned about wait times.

- *If multiple focus groups on the same topic are well moderated, they will yield similar findings.* The reality is that if people were consistent and predictable, we would not have to assemble multiple focus groups or perform much of the surveying currently done in health care. The purpose of focus groups is not to attain unanimity but rather to glean insights from the participants.
- *The time of day when a focus group is held is immaterial.* The reality is that the times when focus groups are conducted will often determine their composition. Focus groups held during the day, for instance, will probably exclude most working people while attracting a high percentage of retirees. The optimal time to conduct focus groups is in the early evening hours.
- *Some type of remuneration or gift should always be given to participants to encourage attendance.* The reality is that many health care providers have gathered participants for focus groups without offering any type of gift or payment. People are generally interested enough in their health care that they will participate without any extrinsic rewards. It can also be argued that an expensive gift may predispose participants to be less critical of their health care provider. Generally, a token gift is offered to participants, such as a hospital T-shirt, coffee mug, or complimentary meal.

For a concise, yet comprehensive, overview of how to use focus groups for market research, see R. A. Krueger's *Focus Groups: A Practical Guide for Applied Research.*[18]

Conclusion

The service elements of health care are very important to the public. When consumers in Oregon were asked to judge the importance of various health plan performance measures, they viewed patient satisfaction measures as one of the most useful indicators of quality.[19] However, many aspects of technical quality of care cannot be evaluated by the public. For this reason, satisfaction ratings as well as other service-related quality measures will continue to influence the consumer's choice of providers for quite some time.

Several basic steps are involved in collecting quantitative data using a health care satisfaction survey. The process should begin with establishing clear expectations for the survey information and how it will be used. Next, concepts should be determined and questions selected. After constructing the survey instrument, it should be tested for validity. And after the survey has been administered, its results should be analyzed. A popular means of obtaining qualitative data is the focus group. Focus groups permit discussion of a range of health topics and work best when the goals for the research are well defined and specific. These concepts can be used to collect and report meaningful data to the public.

References

1. Agency for Health Care Policy and Research, Center for Health Information Dissemination, "AHCPR and Kaiser Examine Consumers' Use of Quality Information," *Research Activities,* no. 199 (December 1996): 10–11.

2. R. Bergman, "Making the Grade," *Hospitals & Health Networks* 68, no. 1 (January 5, 1994): 34–36.

3. M. Gold and J. Wooldridge, "Surveying Consumer Satisfaction to Assess Managed Care Quality: Current Practices," *Health Care Financing Review* 15, no. 4 (summer 1995): 155–73.

4. Agency for Health Care Policy and Research, *Consumer Assessment of Health Plans (CAHPS): Fact Sheet,* publication no. 97-R079 (Rockville, MD: AHCPR, 1997).

5. S. Moretz, "Accreditation '99 Clarifies Rankings," *Managed Healthcare* 8, no. 9 (September 1998): 27–32.

6. F. G. Abdellah and E. Levine, "Developing a Measure of Patient and Personnel Satisfaction with Nursing Care," *Nursing Research* 5 (1957): 100–108.

7. C. E. Rice, D. G. Berger, S. L. Klet, L. G. Sewal, and P.V. Lemkaw, "The Ward Evaluation Scale," *Journal of Clinical Psychology* 19 (1963): 252–60.

8. C. S. Houston and W. E. Pasanen, "Patients' Perceptions of Hospital Care," *Hospitals* 46 (1972): 70–74.

9. J. E. Ware Jr., "Effects of Acquiescent Response Set on Patient Satisfaction Ratings," *Medical Care* 16 (1978): 327–36.

10. S. Strasser and R. M. Davis, *Measuring Patient Satisfaction for Improved Patient Services* (Ann Arbor, MI: Health Administration Press, 1991), pp. 3–25.

11. D. M. Radosevich and T. L. K. Werni, *A Practical Guidebook for Implementing, Analyzing, and Reporting Outcomes Measures* (Bloomington, MN: Stratis Health, 1997), p. 52.

12. F. Fowler, *Improving Survey Questions* (Thousand Oaks, CA: Sage Publications, 1995).

13. W. J. Krowinski and S. R. Steiber, *Measuring and Managing Patient Satisfaction,* 2d ed. (Chicago: American Hospital Publishing, 1996), pp. 187–88.

14. S. Strasser and R. M. Davis, *Measuring Patient Satisfaction for Improved Patient Services* (Ann Arbor, MI: Health Administration Press, 1991), pp.175–98.

15. W. J. Krowinski and S. R. Steiber, *Measuring and Managing Patient Satisfaction,* 2d ed. (Chicago: American Hospital Publishing, 1996), p. 196.

16. D. M. Radosevich and T. L. K. Werni, *A Practical Guidebook for Implementing, Analyzing, and Reporting Outcomes Measures* (Bloomington, MN: Stratis Health, 1997), p. 64.

17. Larry Sachs, senior statistician, Research Department, Healthcare Research Systems, interview with author, Columbus, OH, January 22, 1998.

18. R. A. Krueger, *Focus Groups: A Practical Guide for Applied Research* (Thousand Oaks, CA: Sage Publications, 1994).

19. J. H. Hibbard and J. J. Jewett, "Will Quality Report Cards Help Consumers?" *Health Affairs* 16, no. 3 (March 1997): 218–28.

CHAPTER SEVEN

Assessing How Provider Health Care Programs Enhance Community Quality of Life

Don R. Rahtz, PhD

M. Joseph Sirgy, PhD

Today's health care organizations provide a very broad and integrated system of total prevention and treatment options for consumers. These programs benefit the entire community served by the health care system. By improving people's health status, increasing access to care, and wisely managing health care resources, providers are making a significant social contribution. To be effective, providers must communicate their quality performance to their customers, and their assessments of performance must be guided by valid measures. These measures should reflect the provider's emphasis on a community-based value.

This chapter presents a dynamic, strategic tool for measuring a health care organization's contribution to the community. This instrument can be used to gather subjective data that measure the value of health care services in terms of the community's quality of life. By combining the results of this assessment with the financial data now being used to measure community benefits, health care systems will be able to effectively communicate to the public the value of their social contributions.

Experiments with Measuring and Communicating Provider Health Plan Benefits

A variety of groups are experimenting with methods to quantify and communicate the community benefits offered by health care providers. Many health systems report these benefits in terms of financial contributions. For example, in 1996 College Station Medical Center, a for-profit hospital in College Station, Texas, reportedly provided charity care and government-sponsored indigent health care services in an amount equal to 4.6 percent of the hospital's net patient revenue.[1] St. Vincent Hospital, a not-for-profit hospital in Santa Fe, New Mexico, has prepared a detailed financial report of its community contributions for fiscal year 1997. This report, available on St. Vincent Hospital's Web site (http://www.stvin.org/overview_community_accountability_report.htm), describes the total estimated dollars contributed in benefits to the broader community in five areas: clinic/primary care services, health education, counseling, family services, and in-kind donations. The expenditures on benefits for the poor (Medicaid patient care and medically indigent care) are also reported.

The Michigan Health & Hospital Association gathered financial data as well as numbers of people served by Michigan hospital programs in a 1997 community-benefits survey. The 130 not-for-profit hospitals and health systems that responded to the survey furnished information about the dollar amount of charity and uncompensated care provided and the number of people who benefited from low-cost or free health and wellness programs and services offered by the hospital.[2] The results of this survey were reported to the public in the *Michigan Hospital Report* published in May 1998.

As managed competition continues to evolve, all of the various prevention and treatment programs sponsored by health care systems will be more closely evaluated. It is becoming increasingly clear that financial measures alone do not fully describe the contributions made by a health care system to improve the overall health and welfare of the community it serves. Objective measures of charity and uncompensated care costs and the number of people served by wellness and health education programs do not adequately demonstrate the broader community value of the various elements of the health care system.

Basic Assumptions Regarding Community Satisfaction with Quality of Life

Several factors contribute to the well-being of community residents. Health care services are just one of many elements that influence residents' judgments about the quality of community life. If health care providers are to make claims that their systems have contributed significantly to community residents' well-being, it is crucial that these other factors be recognized and accounted for when measuring the contribution of an individual health care system. Likewise, if people express concerns about the conditions of the community, providers will want to be able to show that the health care system is not at fault.

The basic premise of the community Quality of Life (QOL) Model discussed in this chapter is that life satisfaction is functionally related to satisfaction with all of life's domains and subdomains. That is, life satisfaction is influenced by lower levels of life concerns and evaluations within those levels. The greater the satisfaction with such concerns as personal health, work, family, and leisure, the greater the satisfaction with life in general. In other words, life satisfaction is determined by satisfaction with the mix of an individual's major life domains.

The affect (or feeling) within a life domain spills over vertically (moving up one's set of domains) to the most superordinate domain (life in general), thus determining overall life satisfaction. Satisfaction with a given life domain is determined by satisfaction with life conditions and concerns making up that domain. For example, satisfaction with personal health (a life domain) is determined by satisfaction with community health care satisfaction and one's efforts to eat nutritiously, exercise regularly, drink in moderation, practice safe sex, and so forth.

A person's evaluation of these factors can be viewed as satisfaction/dissatisfaction with life conditions or concerns within the life domain of personal health. Within a given life condition or concern (such as community health care), satisfaction with that life condition or concern is affected by satisfaction with the subconditions (or subconcerns) embedded within it. For example, community health care satisfaction is likely to be determined by satisfaction with the various health care programs and services perceived available in the community (for example, alcohol and drug abuse programs, elderly health services, home health services, inpatient hospital services, outpatient hospital services). These are subconditions/subconcerns embedded hierarchically within the life condition/concern of community health care. The extent to which satisfaction within a subdomain affects satisfaction of a superordinate domain in the hierarchy of psychological domains has been referred to in the QOL literature as the bottom–up spillover effect.[3]

Based on the same theoretical rationale, the following assumptions are articulated concerning the consequences of community health care satisfaction:

- Assumption 1: Community health care satisfaction is a direct function of the sum of satisfactions with various health care programs and services perceived available in the community. In other words, it is assumed that the global community health care satisfaction measure is directly related to the combination of community member satisfactions with all the programs and services offered in a particular service area.

- Assumption 2: Personal health satisfaction is a direct function of community health care satisfaction.
- Assumption 3: Community satisfaction is a direct function of community health care satisfaction.
- Assumption 4: Life satisfaction is a direct function of personal health satisfaction, community satisfaction, job satisfaction, and family satisfaction.

What does all this really mean? It means that health care providers must have a way to track specific contributions its various system elements make to the community and its residents. To do this, they need a means by which to measure those elements.

Quality of Life Model

Although a theoretical model may appear to be the "academic and not real-world" side of things, it does provide an important road map for managers to use in conceptualizing, strategizing, implementing, and monitoring the performance of services. With the growth of prevention programs and integration of primary care networks into the system, health care organizations now offer a wide variety of health care programs and services, and the QOL Model can help managers visualize how all these components fit together in the measurement process.

The QOL Model itself is quite extensive and reflects the complexities of today's environment. (See figure 7-1.) Use of such a model provides a specific framework in which to examine the entire range of health care needs of a community. It allows an evaluation of the extent to which specific health care services and programs (from a given provider) can significantly contribute

Figure 7-1. The QOL Model

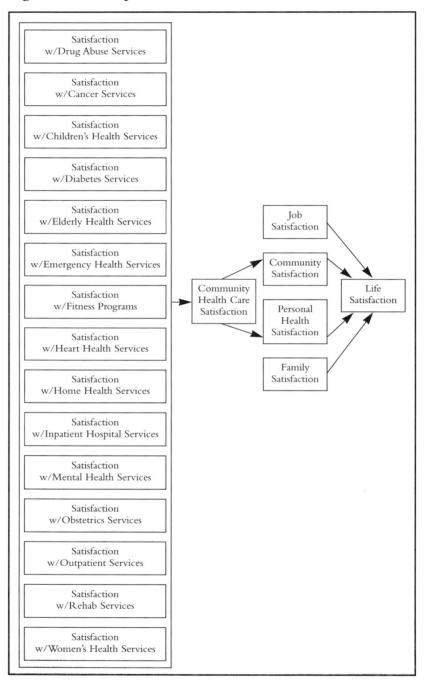

to the quality of life of the community. Although the model is quite comprehensive, it does allow health care managers to distinguish the various components of the health care system. Each of the elements can be assessed as to its individual value and contribution to community residents' QOL. The components of this model are explored in the following subsections.

Measuring the Model Elements

Each of the elements of the model is easily measured using standard rating scales familiar to any marketing research firm. For the model to be used as a full strategic tool, it is necessary to collect data on all its parts. For tactical application, subcomponents can be selected and used on their own. These elements include the following:

- Community health care satisfaction
- Antecedents of community health care satisfaction
- Outcomes of community health care satisfaction

These elements are discussed in the following subsections.

Community Health Care Satisfaction   Community health care satisfaction refers to an overall or global satisfaction a person may feel toward the general health care environment in his or her community. This assessment can be assumed to be a function of the person's perception of general health care programs and services in the community. These programs or services may include alcohol and drug abuse programs, inpatient hospital care, outpatient hospital care, and elderly health services, among others.

Antecedents of Community Health Care Satisfaction
On the left side of the model's diagram are the health system's potential and actual offerings within a given community. It is important to note here that the offerings can be as few, or as

many, as desired. In addition, elements can be added and sub-tracted with no degradation to the model. The effect of an ele-ment's addition or subtraction on other elements and to the system as a whole, however, can be evaluated. This allows dynamic assessments of the entire portfolio of programs and services. Offerings used in this particular example are shown in figure 7-2.

Outcomes of Community Health Care Satisfaction

Portfolio offerings of the system are then evaluated, individu-ally, by community residents. This evaluation provides a bridge to the assessment of their overall satisfaction with health care in the community (community health care satisfaction). Their overall satisfaction is determined by the sum of the satisfac-tions with those health care programs and services residents perceive as available within the community. Simply stated, a measure of overall community health care satisfaction is cre-ated by combining the community member's satisfaction rat-ing for all the relevant elements. In a formula representation, that relationship is expressed as:

$$CHCS = \sum_{i=1}^{n} S_i$$

where:

CHCS = Community *Health Care Satisfaction*

$\sum_{i=1}^{n} S_i$ = Satisfaction with an individual health care program or service i (for example, alcohol and drug abuse programs), where i = 1, 2, 3, 4, . . . , n (n = all the programs/services)

What must be recognized is that respondents may be rating actual or potential health care services and programs provided by one or more health care providers in the community. Consumers can express dissatisfaction with a particular health care program or service that is lacking in the community, as well as those

Figure 7-2. Potential Health Care Programs and Services in a Community

• Alcohol and drug abuse programs	• Home health services
• Cancer services	• Inpatient hospital services
• Children's health services	• Mental health services
• Diabetes services	• Obstetrics services
• Elderly health services	• Outpatient hospital services
• Emergency health services	• Physical rehabilitation services
• Physical fitness programs	• Women's health services
• Heart disease services	

already established. Hence, the list of programs and services that can be included in a community health care assessment instrument does not have to be restricted to actual community offerings. Potential health care programs and services can and should be included in the assessment survey to provide strategic input regarding community offerings. In addition, this model allows for programs and services to be added or subtracted from the assessment instrument to remain consistent with the health care system's real or anticipated portfolio changes.

Measuring Satisfaction with Individual Programs and Services

This section discusses the way that health care decision makers can evaluate individual health care programs and services. To help understand this evaluation, a section of the survey instrument related to physical fitness programs and facilities is shown in figure 7-3 and will be used as an example.

As shown in the figure, satisfaction with physical fitness programs and facilities is measured using a multiplicative index covering four components:

1. Perceived importance of the health care service/program in the community

Figure 7-3. Excerpt from the Survey Questionnaire

Physical Fitness Program and Facilities

(These services include wellness/fitness centers, health improvement classes, diet assistance, nutrition, and healthy families.)

1. How **important** are Physical Fitness Programs to you, your family, and friends in the community?

   ____very important ____important ____somewhat important
   ____not very ____not at all

2. How **satisfied** are you with the quality of this health service in your community?

   ____very satisfied ____satisfied ____somewhat satisfied ____not very
   ____not at all

3. Have you, your family, or friends **used** Physical Fitness Programs/ Facilities in the area in the past?

   ____I have used ____A family member has used
   ____A friend has used
   ____I do not know of anyone who has used this service.

   If the service was used, generally, which area facility/system did you or family/friend use?

   ____Provider #1 ____Provider #2 ____Provider #3 ____Provider #4
   ____Provider #5 ____Other (please specify) _____

   (Note: In the actual survey, the full names of local area providers would be listed above.)

   If this service was used, generally, what is the name of the doctor or provider that you or family/friend use?

   (Please fill in the provider/doctor's name) _____
   ____Don't know

4. How much **knowledge** do you have about this health service in your community?

   ____A great deal ____A good amount ____I have some
   ____I have very little ____I have none

Comments: _____

2. Satisfaction with the quality of the health care service/ program in the community
3. Past use of the health care service/program in the community
4. Knowledge of availability of the health care service/program in the community

Respondent answers to these questions are combined to create an overall satisfaction score. This conception is represented by the formula illustrated in figure 7-4. Each of the provider's community health care programs and services can be measured using these four index components.

The multiplicative nature of the index was developed based on the notion that information gathered from community members must be considered within the context of certain restraints and logic. For example, if someone has firsthand knowledge of a program, the weight given to that individual's assessment should, by logic, be greater than that of an individual who assesses based on second- or thirdhand knowledge. In addition, it is easy to understand that if a service has little or no importance to an individual, that service will play a much smaller role in his or her assessment of overall health

Figure 7-4. Formula for Measuring Service Satisfaction

$$S = Q \times I \times U \times K$$

Where:

S = Satisfaction with the community health care program/service in question
Q = Satisfaction with the quality of the community health care program/service in question
I = Perceived importance of the health care service/program in question within the community
U = Past use of the health care program/service in question within the community
K = Knowledge of the availability of the health service/program in question in the community

care service satisfaction than a service that is of high importance. The index components are multiplied together to arrive at an overall satisfaction score. This is described in greater detail below.

Quality   The focus here is not objective quality of a given health care program, but its perceived quality (Q). For example, how does the resident respondent perceive the quality of the health care program in question? As shown in figure 7-3, satisfaction with the quality of the health care services/programs in question can be measured by responses to the following question: "How satisfied are you with the quality of this health service in your community?" Responses can be tapped on a scale involving five categories: "very satisfied," "satisfied," "somewhat satisfied," "not very," and "not at all." "Very satisfied" responses are coded as +2, "satisfied" as +1, "somewhat satisfied" as −1, "not very" as −2, and "not at all" as −3.

Importance   Because the focus here is to predict community health care satisfaction and not overall satisfaction with an individual health care component, the perceived importance should be construed and measured at a higher level of analysis (the health care service/program in question instead of the attribute level). Therefore, the perceived importance (I, as shown in figure 7-4) is measured by asking respondents the importance of the health care service/program in question in relation to other health care programs and services within the community.

As shown in figure 7-3, perceived importance of the health care service/program in question can be measured by responses to the following question: "How important is this [name of the health care program or service] to you, your family, and friends in the community?" Responses can be tapped on a scale involving five categories: "very important," "important," "somewhat important," "not very," and "not at all." "Very important" responses are coded as 1.0, "important" as .8, "somewhat important" as .6, "not very" as .4, and "not at all" as .2.

Usage and Knowledge Besides perceived importance, it is expected that satisfaction with the quality of a health care service/program will be moderated by the extent of the consumer's use of the health care service/program in question, as well as his or her knowledge of its availability. The greater the use (U) of the service or program in question, the more intense the satisfaction with the quality of the service or program. Similarly, the greater the knowledge (K) of the availability of the service or program in question, the more intense is the resultant satisfaction.

As shown in figure 7–3, past use of the health care service/program in question can be measured by responses to the following response cue: "Have you, your family, or friend used [name of the health care program or service] in the area in the past?" This statement should be followed by four response categories: "I have used" (coded as 1.00), "A family member has used" (coded as .85), "A friend has used" (coded as .50), "I do not know of anyone who used this service" (coded as .25).

Knowledge of the availability of the health care service/program in question can be measured by responses to the following question: "How much knowledge do you have about this [health service] in your community?" Responses can be tapped on a scale involving five categories: "a great deal," "a good amount," "I have some," "I have very little," and "I have none." "A great deal" responses are coded as 1.0, "a good amount" as .8, "I have some" as .6, "I have very little" as .4, and "I have none" as .2.

Satisfaction Satisfaction (S) with the community health care program/service in question is not measured directly by a specific question. Instead, it is measured as a composite of respondents' perception of quality (Q) of the program/service, its importance (I) in relation to other health care programs and services, the extent of use (U) of the program/service, and the knowledge (K) the respondent has about it. Therefore, each respondent has a composite score computed by multiplying Q with I, U, and K.

Measuring Community Health Care Satisfaction

Community health care satisfaction refers to residents' overall feelings of satisfaction with the various health care programs and services available in the community. It can be measured by responses to the following question: "In general, how satisfied are you with the overall quality of the health care available in this area?" Responses are recorded using the Delighted–Terrible scale.[4] This scale has been well validated in a wide number of studies. The specific categories are: "delighted" (coded as 7), "pleased" (coded as 6), "mostly satisfied" (coded as 5), "mixed or equally satisfied and dissatisfied" (coded as 4), "mostly dissatisfied" (coded as 3), "unhappy" (coded as 2), "terrible" (coded as 1), "neutral or neither satisfied nor dissatisfied" (coded as missing data), and "never thought about it" (coded as missing data).

Measuring Other Community and Global Life Domains

Community satisfaction, personal health satisfaction, job satisfaction, family satisfaction, and life satisfaction are all measured using the Delighted–Terrible scale. Specifically, community satisfaction can be measured by responses to the following question: "Overall, how satisfied are you with the community in which you live?" For personal health satisfaction: "Overall, how do you feel about your personal health at this time?" For job satisfaction: "Overall, how satisfied are you in general with your job?" For family satisfaction: "Overall, how satisfied are you with your family?" And finally, life satisfaction should be measured by responses to the following question: "Overall, how satisfied are you with your life?"

How to Apply the QOL Model and Method

The QOL model has been used in various pilot studies and was recently used in conducting an assessment for a regional health care system. Based on the authors' preparatory work and the full-scale application, several methodological and application recommendations can be made. It is suggested that health care organizations conduct the first study in four interrelated phases:

1. Preliminary interviews
2. Telephone-screening survey
3. Survey instrument development
4. Main survey collection

The process can be adjusted in follow-up studies.

Phase 1: Preliminary Interviews

Phase 1 consists of personal interviews with community health care providers, as well as community leaders, to identify the types of health care programs that are available in the community. (For example, in our study the interview with the vice-president of programs of the health care organization in question identified the following programs and services: drug abuse, cancer, diabetes, elderly, emergency, fitness, heart, home health, inpatient, mental health, obstetrics, outpatient, rehabilitation, and women's health.) The initial survey instrument is developed after an assessment of these interviews. Any study specification or application problems that can be identified at this point will save a significant amount of time, effort, and money during the main survey collection phase.

Phase 2: Telephone-Screening Survey

Phase 2 is a telephone-screening survey to identify a group of respondents for use in the full study in Phase 4. Although other methods for identifying study participants can be used, the telephone survey provides a quick turnaround and can be done at minimal cost. For example, to select approximately 400 people for the main study sample, more than 500 individuals should be contacted using a probabilistic sampling procedure from the area telephone book or other readily available database.

The telephone-screening interview should not take more than five minutes to complete. Here respondents are asked about their demographics and a few questions about the quality of the area's health care. At the end of that survey, respondents are asked if they would be willing to participate in a much more detailed mail survey concerning health care offerings in the community. The provider might consider offering some incentive (for example, a lottery of a cash prize such as $1,000) to encourage participation.

Phase 3: Survey Instrument Development

Due to space constraints, a full presentation of the survey instrument used in recent studies is not included in this chapter. In lieu of seeing the entire instrument, a brief narrative of the survey elements follows. The total length of the questionnaire should not exceed ten pages. The following subsections focus on developing and pretesting the questionnaire content.

Introductory Section   The survey questionnaire is entitled "Your Opinions on Community Health Care." Instruction, such as the following, is provided at the beginning of the questionnaire:

> This questionnaire seeks to gain a better understanding of Community X residents' opinions about the local heath care service. When answering, please remember your opinions are very important to us, so please be as truthful as possible. Your answers will help in designing better health care programs for your community.

It is important in the introductory comments to stress the value that the individual will gain by participating in the study.

Placement Order and Formatting Issues The measure for community health care satisfaction should be placed at the beginning of the questionnaire, followed by the measures pertaining to personal health satisfaction, community satisfaction, job satisfaction, family satisfaction, and life satisfaction. Ordering is important to minimize potential bias. Between these questions should be filler questions designed to reduce other response biases. For example, questions pertaining to ratings of physical health along a variety of dimensions can be used as fillers.

With respect to the measures pertaining to the individual health care programs and services, figure 7–3 (the instrument portion included in the questionnaire) offers formatting suggestions. This portion of the questionnaire should begin with clear instructions. These are the critical portfolio assessment data, and it is important that everyone is clear on how to respond. The introductory statement might read as follows:

> The following set of questions asks you about a wide variety of health services and programs that are offered in community X by a number of health care providers. Each particular service has a number of questions that relate to that particular service. We would like to know your feelings on how important it is that the service is available, how satisfied you are with the particular type of service, and any experience you, your family, or friends may have had. Please answer these questions as they relate to you personally or to your family and friends. Your answers will be very useful in making any changes you think are necessary for better community health care.

Demographics The last portion of the questionnaire should involve demographic items. Early in the survey people are less likely to respond to personal items. Be sure to include all relevant demographics. For example, zip codes are an easy and important data element to obtain. In addition, performance of the system in serving at-risk populations can be partitioned out through the use of age, ethnicity, income, and other types of variables.

Pretesting   The survey instrument to be used in the main study should be pretested on a small sample of residents (for example, ten residents). Discussions should follow the administration of the instrument to adjust wording and layout. The revised instrument can then be mailed to the individuals who expressed a willingness to participate. It is also suggested that a focus group drawn from the sample be involved in a "poststudy" assessment. This assessment can provide a wealth of information on areas of interest, as well as a check on the entire study process.

Phase 4: Main Survey Collection

The survey instrument is mailed to the individuals who expressed a willingness to participate in the study. Expect an approximate response rate of 25 percent. Thus, a mailing of 400 questionnaires will likely result in a return of 100 completed ones. Most people in the community are concerned about health care, but oversurveying by various marketing research firms has left many people wary of responding.

How to Analyze Survey Results

Analyzing the results from the data collection can be as simple or as complex as you want it to be. On the one hand, simple assessments of mean scores, or even frequencies of satisfaction measures, can provide insight into performance. Moving to more complex analysis can provide a much more extensive wealth of strategic applications. In either case, the main appeal of the QOL measurement approach is in its integrative capability, making it easy to see how the various elements of the system interact with each other and the rest of the environment. Should readers wish additional detailed information on how the model's results can be analyzed with inferential and descriptive statistic tests, they are encouraged to contact the authors directly.[5]

The information gained from the study can be disseminated both internally and externally. The data from the process can be used internally throughout the organization as performance baselines and for strategic planning purposes. This same information, in a more general form, can be shared with interested external stakeholders (the community, public officials, and so on) to demonstrate the health care system's contribution to the betterment of the community.

How to Apply Study Results

How can health care providers use this assessment method to enhance the quality of life of community residents? Each program or service can simply be evaluated on the basis of the mean scores or frequency reports. More complex statistical analysis can be used to test each of the research assumptions presented earlier in this chapter. Advanced analysis techniques can be used to determine the overall effect of satisfaction with the various health care programs and services on people's life satisfaction.

Probably the easiest way to illustrate the application of the data is to describe how the information has been used in the past by a health care organization. The discussion centers on posing a performance-related question, interpreting the statistics, and providing some recommendations on possible actions that could be taken. The data in table 7-1 showing means and standard deviations of measures of satisfaction with individual health care services will be used in this example. Following are examples of questions to ask:

1. Which health care services in the community are lacking in quality? Based on the figures in table 7-1, most community residents report dissatisfaction with health care programs and services related to elderly health (mean of satisfaction w/quality = $-9.\text{E-}02$), alcohol and drug abuse

Table 7-1. Means and Standard Deviations of Measures of Satisfaction with Individual Health Care Services

Health Service	Satisfaction w/Quality	Perceived Importance	Use	Knowledge
Women's health	.57 (1.22)	.95 (.11)	.85 (.25)	.72 (.19)
Children's health	.68 (1.13)	.97 (7.54E-02)	.75 (.31)	.68 (.21)
Elderly health	−9.E-02 (1.27)	.91 (.14)	.52 (.27)	.57 (.21)
Physical fitness	.27 (1.25)	.84 (.16)	.61 (.30)	.67 (.19)
Outpatient	.82 (1.11)	.94 (.11)	.83 (.24)	.72 (.18)
Cancer	.34 (1.13)	.95 (.11)	.47 (.25)	.61 (.21)
Alcohol/drug abuse	−7.E-02 (1.3)	.90 (.14)	.40 (.22)	.58 (.20)
Heart disease	.66 (1.15)	.94 (.10)	.59 (.29)	.63 (.21)
Diabetes	.28 (1.11)	.89 (.14)	.42 (.24)	53 (.21)
Obstetrics	.90 (.99)	.94 (.10)	.72 (.29)	.70 (.21)
Physical rehab.	.41 (1.11)	.88 (.15)	.49 (.28)	.55 (.21)
Psychiatric/mental	.11 (1.23)	.89 (.16)	.46 (.27)	.59 (.21)
Home health	−.17 (1.32)	.87 (.16)	.42 (.24)	.54 (.22)
Inpatient	.39 (1.22)	.91 (.13)	.69 (.29)	.67 (.21)
Emergency	.51 (1.28)	.97 (8.66E-02)	.71 (.29)	.70 (.18)

Satisfaction = Satisfaction with the quality of the health care services/program. This was measured by responses to the following question: "How satisfied are you with the quality of this health service in the community?" Responses were tapped on a scale involving five categories: "very satisfied," "satisfied," "somewhat satisfied," "not very," and "not at all." "Very satisfied" responses were coded as +2, "satisfied" as +1, "somewhat satisfied" as −1, "not very" as −2, and "not at all" as −3.

Importance = Perceived importance of the health care service/program. This was measured by responses to the following question: "How important is this [name of the health care program or service] to the community?" Responses were tapped on a scale involving five categories: "very important," "important," "somewhat important," "not very," and "not at all." "Very important" responses were coded as 1.0, "important" as .8, "somewhat important" as .6, "not very" as .4, and "not at all" as .2.

Use = Past use of the health care service/program. This was measured by responses to the following response cue: "Concerning the use of [name of the health care program or service]." This statement was followed by four response categories: "I have used" (coded as 1.0), "A family member has used" (coded as .85), "A friend has used" (coded as .5), "I do not know of anyone who used this service" (coded as .25).

Knowledge = Knowledge of the availability of the health care service/program. This was measured by responses to the following question: "How much knowledge about available [name of the health care program or service] would you say you have?" Responses were tapped on a scale involving five categories: "a large amount," "a fair amount," "some," "very little," and "none." "A large amount" responses were coded as 1.0, "a fair amount" as .8, "some" as .6, "very little" as .4, and "none" as .2.

(mean of satisfaction with quality $= -7.E-02$), and home health (mean of satisfaction with quality $= -.17$). However, it should be noted that there is a disparity of opinions regarding residents' perception of quality of these health care services as noted by their standard deviations (1.27, 1.30, and 1.32, respectively).

2. How important are these health care services to residents of the community? To answer this question, one needs to examine the perceived importance means of these health care services as shown in table 7-1. The majority of residents report that these three types of health care services are "very important" (means of perceived importance = .91, .90, and .87, respectively). This should lead health care providers and public policy officials to realize that these three types of health care services are lacking and are important to the community citizenry.

3. Could the reported dissatisfaction be due to lack of knowledge of the availability of these services? If so, action should be taken to increase the promotional efforts of these services to educate the community residents of their availability. Table 7-1 shows that most community residents have "some" knowledge of these health care services (means of knowledge = .57, .58, and .54, respectively). Perhaps the action necessary here is to increase the promotional efforts to educate the public about the availability of these services in the community.

4. Are the health care services that are identified to be lacking in quality heavily used by the community residents? If so, action should be taken to further develop these services. Table 7-1 shows that most community residents know of friends and acquaintances who have used the aforementioned services (means of use = .52, .40, and .42, respectively). Based on these results, action should be taken to further develop (or at least maintain) health care programs and services related to elderly health, alcohol and drug abuse, and home health.

How to Enhance Community Quality of Life

Ultimately, the value of a health care system is determined by the residents of the community it serves. Therefore, it is important to use this method as a means of building stronger bonds with the community. To do that, make the community aware of your concern for the residents and how your performance contributes to their well-being. This can be accomplished in any number of ways. Publicizing your findings through special events, strategic alliances, community report cards, city council meetings, board of directors meetings, and healthy community group meetings can generate a lot of community support. Effective use of the data can enhance your partnership with the community. For example, by attending (or even organizing) healthy community group meetings, your organization's willingness to be involved beyond the simple delivery of services is clearly evident. Parts of your data can be used by those in attendance to assess how changes might be brought about in the community. A yearly announcement of the "Health of the Community" can highlight progress made by your organization and generate a significant amount of media coverage and community awareness.

However, it is important to be truthful with your results. People can see through a "smoke screen." If there are some negatives in the results (which there always are), they should be disclosed. Research has clearly demonstrated that people are much more likely to "believe" and "identify with" organizations that disclose their shortcomings as well as their strengths. When you show you are "not hiding anything," the improvements you will later make will be all the more gratifying to the community.

Conclusion

The QOL assessment process can increase awareness of your health care programs and performance. By using this survey method on a regular basis, the community can become involved in monitoring performance improvements. There will be a clear recognition that the health care system does contribute value to the broader community. When the provider can demonstrate to the community that it really does use the data it collects on the community's quality of life, the goodwill from such endeavors will be tremendous.

Health care systems must be able to demonstrate their value to the community they serve. The public's perceptions of health care providers is the reality within which organizations must operate. It is these perceptions that influence the actions of lawmakers, public policy officials, and consumer advocacy groups. The value of a tool that aids in monitoring these perceptions is quite clear. From both a strategic and tactical perspective, health care providers can allocate resources and make adjustments to their portfolio of programs and services that will result in the delivery of an optimal product—one that is viewed by the community as having been customized for their needs and that they, as stakeholders, can share in and embrace.

References

1. College Station Medical Center, "Financial Information," WWW document, September 1998, URL: http://www.columbia-bv.com/ services/finance.htm.

2. Michigan Health & Hospital Association, *Michigan Hospital Report* (Lansing, MI: MHA, 1998), pp. 15–22.

3. M. J. Sirgy, "Strategic Marketing Planning Guided by the Quality-of-Life (QOL) Concept," *Journal of Business Ethics* 15, no. 3 (March 1996): 241–59.

4. F. M. Andrews and S. B. Withey, *Social Indicators of Well-Being: Americans' Perceptions of Life Quality* (New York: Plenum Press, 1976).

5. Don R. Rahtz, The College of William and Mary, School of Business Administration, Williamsburg, Virginia 23187, 757-221-2866 (office), 757-221-2937 (fax), dxraht@dogwood.tyler.wm.edu (e-mail), http:// www.swem.wm.edu/class/rahtz.html (personal Web page); M. Joseph Sirgy, Virginia Polytechnic Institute and State University, Department of Marketing, 2025 Pamplin Hall, Blacksburg, Virginia 24061, 540-231-5110 (office), 540-231-3076 (fax), sirgy@st.edu (e-mail), http://www.cob.st.edu/market/faculty/sirgy/personal/sirgy.htm (personal Web page).

Additional Resources

Books

Borgstadt, N., ed. *Get Ready-Get Set-Go-Go-Go: A Marketing Primer for Home Health Care Professionals* (Boston: Visiting Nurse Association of America, 1997).

Cooper, P. D., ed. *Health Care Marketing: A Foundation for Managed Quality* (Gaithersburg, MD: Aspen Publishers, 1994).

Curtis, R., and T. Kurtz. *Creating Consumer Choice in Healthcare: Measuring and Communicating Health Plan Performance Information* (Chicago: Health Administration Press, 1998).

Grenlick, M. R., and P. P. Hanes. *Grading Health Care: The Science and Art of Developing Consumer Scorecards* (San Francisco: Jossey-Bass Publishers, 1998).

Leebov, W., S. Afrait, and J. Presha. *Service Savvy Health Care* (Chicago: AHA Press, 1998).

Leebov, W., G. Scott, and L. Olson, eds. *Achieving Impressive Customer Satisfaction* (Chicago: AHA Press, 1998).

Morrisey, M. A., ed. *Managed Care and Changing Health Care Markets* (Washington, DC: AEI Press, 1997).

Sherman, S. G., and V. C. Sherman. *Total Customer Satisfaction: A Comprehensive Approach for Health Care Providers* (San Francisco: Jossey-Bass Publishers, 1998).

Sturm, A. C. *The New Rules of Healthcare Marketing: 23 Strategies for Success* (Chicago: Health Administration Press, 1998).

Zimmerman, D., P. Zimmerman, and C. Lund, eds. *The Healthcare Customer Revolution: The Growing Impact of Managed Care on Patient Satisfaction* (Westchester, IL: Healthcare Financial Management Association. 1996).

Journal Articles

Aron, D. C., et al. "Impact of Risk-Adjusting Cesarean Delivery Rates When Reporting Hospital Performance," *Journal of the American Medical Association* 279, no. 24 (June 24, 1998): 1968–72.

Edgman-Levitan, S., and P. D. Cleary. "What Information Do Consumers Want and Need?" *Health Affairs* 14, no. 1 (winter 1996): 42–56.

Epstein, A. M. "Rolling Down the Runway: Challenges Ahead for Quality Report Cards," *Journal of the American Medical Association* 279, no. 21 (June 3, 1998): 691–96.

Fergusen, T. "Health Online and the Empowered Medical Consumer," *Joint Commission Journal on Quality Improvement* 23, no. 5 (May 1997): 251–57.

Hibbard, J. H., and E. C. Weeks. "Does the Dissemination of Comparative Data on Physician Fees Affect Consumer Use of Services?" *Medical Care* 27, no. 12 (December 1989): 1167–74.

Hibbard, J. H., and J. J. Jewett. "What Type of Quality Information Do Consumers Want in a Health Care Report Card?" *Medical Care Research and Review* 53, no. 1 (March 1996): 28–47.

Hibbard, J. H., and J. J. Jewett. "Will Quality Report Cards Help Consumers?" *Health Affairs* 16, no. 3 (March 1997): 218–28.

Hibbard, J. H., P. Slovic, and J. J. Jewett. "Informing Consumer Decisions in Health Care: Implications from Decision-Making Research," *Milbank Quarterly* 75, no. 3 (1997): 395–414.

Hibbard, J. H., J. J. Jewett, S. Engelman, and M. Tusler. "Can Medicare Beneficiaries Make Informed Choices?" *Health Affairs* 17, no. 4 (November/December 1998).

Hochhauser, M. "Designing Readable Report Cards," *Managed Healthcare* 8, no. 5 (May 1998): 14–22.

Hopkins, M. S. "Value in Health Care: What Providers and Employers Say," *Healthcare Financial Management* 52, no. 7 (July 1998): 66–70.

Hoy, E. W., E. K. Wicks, and R. A. Forland. "A Guide to Facilitating Consumer Choice," *Health Affairs* 15, no. 1 (winter 1996): 9–30.

Isaacs, S. I. "Consumer's Information Needs: Results of a National Survey," *Health Affairs* 15, no. 1 (winter 1996): 31–41.

Knutson, D. J., J. B. Fowles, M. Finch, J. McGee, N. Dahms, E. A. Kind, and S. Adlis. "Employer-Specific Versus Community-Wide Report Cards: Is There a Difference?" *Health Care Financing Review* 18, no. 1 (fall 1996): 111–25.

MacStravic, S. "Don't Just Deliver Value, Demonstrate It," *Health Care Strategic Management* 16, no. 8 (August 1998): 1, 20–23.

Maloney, S. K., J. Finn, D. L. Bloom, and J. Anderson. "Personal Decision Making Styles and Long-Term Care Choices," *Health Care Financing Review* 18, no. 1 (fall 1996): 141–55.

McGee, J., D. Kanouse, S. Sofaer, L. Hargraves, E. Hoy, and S. Klieman. "Making Survey Results Easy to Report to Consumers: How Reporting Needs Guided Survey Design in CAHPS," *Medical Care* 36, no. 12 (December 1998).

Mennemeyer, S. T., M.A. Morrisey, and L. Z. Howard. "Death and Reputation: How Consumers Acted upon HCFA Mortality Information," *Inquiry* (summer 1997): 117–28.

Mukamel, D. B., and A. I. Mushlin. "Quality of Care Information Makes a Difference: An Analysis of Market Share and Price Changes After Publications of the New York State Cardiac Surgery Mortality Reports," *Medical Care* 36, no. 7 (July 1998): 945–54.

Raymond, A. G. "Giving Consumers the Quality Information They Need," *Quality Letter* 7 (1995): 15–22.

Robinson, S., and M. Brodie. "Understanding the Quality Challenge for Health Consumers," The Kaiser/AHCPR Survey, *Journal of Quality Improvement* 23, no. 5 (May 1997): 239–44.

Sangl, J. A., and L. F. Wolf. "Role of Consumer Information in Today's Health Care System," *Health Care Financing Review* 18, no. 1 (fall 1996): 1–8.

Schneider, E., and A. M. Epstein. "Patient Use of Public Performance Reports: A Survey of Patients Undergoing Cardiac

Surgery," *Journal of the American Medical Association* 279 (May 1998): 1638–42.

Sofaer, S. "How Will We Know If We Got It Right? Aims, Benefits, and Risks of Consumer Information Initiatives," *Journal on Quality Improvement* 23, no. 5 (May 1997b): 258–64.

Spath, P. L. "Nursing Performance Measures Go Public," *Outcomes Management for Nursing Practice* 2, no. 3 (1998): 10–14.

Spath, P. L. "Taking the Message Public: Presenting Health Quality Information to Consumers," chapter 8 in *1998 Medical Quality Management Sourcebook,* J. Mangano, ed. (New York: Faulkner & Gray, 1997).

Varner, T., and J. Christy, "Consumer Information Needs in a Competitive Health Care Environment," *Health Care Financing Review* (annual supplement 1986): 99–104.

Woodbury, D., et al. "Does Considering Severity of Illness Improve Interpretation of Patient Satisfaction Data?" *Journal for Healthcare Quality* 20, no. 4 (July/August 1998): 33–40.

Zabloki, E. "Are You Providing the Information Purchasers and Consumers Need to Make Informed Decisions?" *Quality Letter* 7 (1995): 2–14.

Other Publications

Agency for Health Care Policy and Research. "Consumer Assessments of Health Plans Study" (CAHPS), AHCPR publication no. 96-R068. April 29, 1996.

"Information: What Do Consumers Have a Right to Have?" Subcommittee on Consumer Rights, Protections and Responsibilities of the Advisory Commission on Consumer

Protection and Quality in the Health Care Industry, Internet, http://www.hcqualitycommission.gov/july21.22/papinfo.htm, printed September 15, 1997.

"President's Advisory Commission on Consumer Protection and Quality in the Health Care Industry." Home page and links, http://www.hcqualitycommission.gov, printed November 19, 1997.

Simmons, H. E. "The Nation's Least Understood Health Care Problem—The Quality of Medical Care," *Generations Magazine* (summer 1996), WWW document URL: http://www. nchc.org/simmons.html.

United States General Accounting Office. "Health Care Employers and Individual Consumers Want Additional Information on Quality." GAO/HEHS-95-201. Report to the Ranking Minority Member, Committee on Labor and Human Resources, U.S. Senate. Washington, DC, 1995.

United States General Accounting Office. "Health Care Reform: 'Report Cards' Are Useful But Significant Issues Need to be Addressed." GAO/HEHS-94-219. Report to the Chairman, Committee on Labor and Human Resources, U. S. Senate. Washington, DC, 1994.

Index